Life Lessons for Women

Jack Canfield
Mark Victor Hansen
Stephanie Marston, M.F.T.

"Life is for Living"

Vermilion

We would like to acknowledge the many publishers and individuals who granted us permission to reprint the cited material. (Note: The stories that were penned anonymously, that are in the public domain or that were written by Jack Canfield, Mark Victor Hansen or Stephanie Marston, M.F.T. are not included in this listing.)

The Love Letter. Reprinted by permission of Deborah Shouse. ©2002 Deborah Shouse.

The Wisdom of the Birds. Reprinted by permission of Susan Siersma. ©2002 Susan Siersma.

With a Little Help from a Stranger. Reprinted by permission of Beadrin E. Youngdahl. ©2002 Beadrin E. Youngdahl.

(Continued on page 293)

1 3 5 7 9 10 8 6 4 2

First published in the United States in 2004 by Health Communications, Inc.

First published in the United Kingdom in 2005 by Vermilion, an imprint of Ebury Publishing
Random House UK Ltd.
Random House, 20 Vauxhall Bridge Road, London SW1V 2SA

Random House Australia (Pty) Limited
20 Alfred Street, Milsons Point, Sydney, New South Wales 2061, Australia

Random House New Zealand Limited
18 Poland Road, Glenfield, Auckland 10, New Zealand

Random House (Pty) Limited
Endulini, 5a Jubilee Road, Parktown 2193, South Africa

Random House UK Limited Reg. No. 954009
www.randomhouse.co.uk
Papers used by Vermilion are natural, recyclable products made from wood grown in sustainable forests.

A CIP catalogue record for this book is available from the British Library

ISBN 0091902592

Printed and bound in Great Britain by Mackays of Chatham plc, Chatham, Kent

Contents

Essential Ingredient #3: Take Care of Yourself

Essential Ingredient #4: Surround Yourself With Support

Introduction

Life Lessons for Women is the first book in a new line of *Chicken Soup* books. It is a true self-help book. We wanted to take the inspiration from the stories in the original *Chicken Soup* series and give you practical tools, exercises and information to support you in creating greater balance, love, health and joy in your life.

Over the years we have received tens of thousands of letters from you, our readers, expressing gratitude, sharing how a particular story affected you or asking for advice. This book is our effort to further provide the support and encouragement you've come to rely on from *Chicken Soup*.

Whether you're a stay-at-home mom managing a household, a career woman balancing work and family, a single mom who is trying to fill in all the gaps or a woman who is simply tired of being tired, *Life Lessons for Women: 7 Essential Ingredients for a Balanced Life* will unveil sensible secrets that will help you to value yourself, savor everyday experiences and find time to live with more joy, vitality and peace in the midst of a chaotic world. It will provide you with the keys to find balance and fulfillment in your complicated, stressful life.

The book is divided into seven Essential Ingredients. Each chapter contains the *Chicken Soup* stories you know and love; Life Lessons that draw out the best of each story; Basic Tools that contain suggestions that can support you in putting the lessons into practice; inspirational quotes; sidebars called Food for Thought and Questions Worth Asking that give you something further to ponder; and The Finishing Touch exercises to help you incorporate what you've just learned. All of these elements are designed to help you connect to what matters most to you, make conscious choices about how you invest your time and energy, and improve the quality of your everyday life.

It is obvious from your e-mails and letters that most of you struggle to focus on yourself, your needs and your dreams. Much of your value has come from your ability to understand other people's needs and to fulfill them. It's one of your talents as women. Yet many of you want to bring yourself back into the equation. You want to begin to attend to your long neglected or forgotten needs and longings. You want to reinstate yourself at the center of your own life. But in order for this to happen, you need to learn to balance your responsibilities to others with responsibility to yourself, obligations with enjoyment, work with play, activity with rest.

When you begin to remember what's most important in your life, when you rekindle your hopes and dreams, when you recommit to your deeply held values and beliefs, you will rediscover your deepest yearnings and recover your joy, wisdom, passion, enthusiasm, self-confidence and vitality—then you can create the life you were truly meant to live.

Life Lessons is a gift from us to you. It will help you rediscover your strengths, and recognize what you love and what you long for. It will show you how to transform your life one essential ingredient at a time. It was created to inspire you to find greater balance and fulfillment, and to reconnect with your passion. Whatever you've been longing to do, whatever you've been yearning to reclaim, now is the time.

It is with this in mind that we offer you *Life Lessons for Women*. May you experience the inspiration, support and encouragement you need to become the joyful, amazing woman you were meant to be.

Jack Canfield, Mark Victor Hansen
and *Stephanie Marston*

RE-COLLECT YOURSELF

Love yourself first and everything else falls into line. You really have to love yourself to get anything done in this world.

Lucille Ball

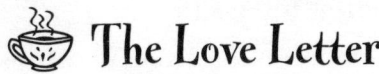 The Love Letter

I must undertake to love myself and to respect myself as though my very life depends upon self-love and self-respect.

JUNE JORDAN

"I want you to write yourself a love letter," the instructor cooed. "Close your eyes and see yourself as the most glorious person in the world. You are the ultimate beloved. Now open your eyes and write."

I shifted in the wooden chair. I had signed up for a two-hour class in "Happiness," and I felt bombarded by positive pushiness, arch affirmations and bliss bombs. Already I had dutifully trooped into the bathroom, looked in the mirror and assured myself that I was beautiful. I tried not to notice that pimple lurking on my nose, the wrinkles wandering from my eyes, or the gorgeous blond next to me, whispering ardently (and truthfully) to herself, "You are so beautiful."

"You're not writing," the teacher scolded. I sighed and rummaged in my purse for scrap paper. On the back of a grocery store receipt, I wrote: "Dear Deborah, You need more time alone. Why are you constantly signing up for self-help classes? Get a grip. Yours, D."

I put down my pen and looked at my watch. *Only fifty-six more minutes of Happiness.* Once home, I reached into the mailbox, pulled out a clump of white envelopes and thought: *Wouldn't it be great if one of these envelopes held a real love letter, from an inconsolable former lover, a secret admirer or a contrite ex-husband?*

The mail was full of passions, pleadings and promises. A credit card company assured me that charging with them meant recharging the world. A long distance carrier swore if I would "go the distance" with them I would save money. A book club promised I could turn over a new leaf if I would just turn into one of their subscribers.

There was no piece of paper that hinted at the intriguing tint of my eyes or the vibrant color of my hair, no mention of the musicality of my voice or the tenderness of my touch.

The more I thought about it, the more appealing a love letter seemed. I brewed a cup of tea, sat at the kitchen table and mentally surveyed the terrain: my partner might fax me a loving quote, e-mail me a fond memo or leave me a sexy voice mail. But I knew no man who would write me a love letter.

So I decided to write one to myself. First, I put on some Johnny Mathis music, dribbled Obsession on my neck and lit the only candle I could find: a thin green birthday candle, which I wedged into a piece of seven-grain bread. Then I closed my eyes, hummed along with "Chances Are" and tried to remember the things I loved about myself. I felt as if I were wearing high heels I could barely walk in.

What were the words my high school hero used in his effusive love letter, written after our first kiss? "You are the most real girl I know." Or the note my college crush had penned: "You are the only girl I will ever love." I wonder if he later repeated the promise to each of his three wives.

"Say whatever comes out," I encouraged myself, like the teacher had urged. I scribbled a few lines on the back of an old envelope, then decided, just this once, I would use some of the beautiful seashell-colored stationery I had bought for some mythical beloved. My hand was sweaty as I picked up my favorite pen.

"Dear Deborah," I wrote, "I admire the way you help other people. I know how hard you try and how much you worry about being good enough. Deborah, you are a good person. Yours, D."

I read the letter and frowned. It sounded like the Boy Scout Pledge meets Co-Dependents Anonymous. Surely, there was a Lady Godiva, an Anna Karenina, an Anaïs Nin somewhere inside me.

I unearthed some magenta nail polish and shined up my

fingernails. I pouted my mouth into BlissBerry Crimson lipstick. I poised my pen over the paper and my mind went blank. So I sat there until Johnny Mathis ran out of songs.

Then I called a former boyfriend, who I knew was between lovers. "What did we used to fight about?" I asked him, after I had inquired about the health and well-being of his prized vintage MG.

"You wanted more attention. I wasn't romantic or punctual enough for you. There was some other stuff, but I've forgotten. Did I tell you I painted her forest green? You should see her in starlight."

I had definitely seen her in starlight way too many times. I hung up and wrote, "Dear Deborah, You are better than any car. You are romantic and always show up on time. I can take you anywhere and never have any problems parking you."

Now I knew why the bookstores sold hardback collections of the world's great love letters. If they were all this difficult to pen, there couldn't be very many of them. I paced the room, determined to write at least a postcard's worth of love.

"Dear Deborah, You have a great sense of humor. You never give up and you are about as cute, smart and creative as you are ever going to be. Enjoy every amazing moment, you succulent creature. Love, Me."

Ahh, this was more romantic. I felt a flutter of

excitement as I reread that letter. I remembered my vow to be in love with life and enjoy every day.

I have a box where I save wonderful things people have written to me. I put my love letter in it. I flopped on the sofa, feeling glamorous and wanted. Oh sure, I knew a day would come, possibly even tomorrow, when the afterglow of the love letter would diminish, when I couldn't think of what was right in my life. Then I would reach into my box, and along with notes from lovers, friends and family, I would find the seashell paper and the words from the toughest, strictest, most exacting person I know. I would find that incredible challenge: "Love Me."

Deborah Shouse

LIFE LESSON #1:
TAKE STOCK OF YOUR LIFE

Most of you long for something more—more time, more money, more friends, a better relationship with your spouse or family. How many times have you heard yourself say, "I wish I had more time for myself"? "This stress is killing me." "I have to exercise and get in better shape." "I want my life to be more fun." "How am I going to make ends meet?" "Where has the day gone? I feel like I haven't gotten anything done!" Sound familiar?

Whether you're a stay-at-home mom managing a household, a working mother balancing work and family, a single mom trying to keep her head above water or a woman who's simply tired of feeling like she's living a "treadmill existence," you have a choice—you can create a life you love.

The first step in doing this is to look back over your life, not with a critical eye, but rather to discover the connecting thread that gives your life rhythm and meaning. In recalling our lives we re-collect ourselves. We gather together our forgotten priorities and passions. Yet in order to do this you have to know who you are and what truly matters.

To love oneself is the beginning of a life-long romance.

Oscar Wilde

You have to ask, what do I love? What are my core values and beliefs? What are my own needs and desires? How can I create a life that fits exactly who I am now, not who I've been? This understanding will provide you with a chance for reevaluation and, if need be, for course corrections.

I appreciate and value myself, for I have done extraordinary things.

☕ Wisdom of the Birds

After raising three children to adulthood, my husband and I were sharing more time together, and we believed that we would have "money in the bank" some day in the not too distant future. "Won't it be great when we're retired?" became a frequent sentence in our conversations. Then, an unforgettable year arrived and changed everything.

It was one of those years, the kind when I found my inner voice whispering, "What else can go wrong?" My mom's health was rapidly failing and our unwed daughter had moved back in with us after delivering a baby girl. During the previous winter, my husband's mother died a slow, cruel death from Alzheimer's disease and his father had been hospitalized following emergency surgery. My husband's mental and physical health began deteriorating with the weight of life's troubles. Our friends and relatives seemed to be experiencing their unfair share of hardships too. Then September 11th happened. Suddenly, my husband's seemingly secure job became very insecure as the economy wavered. Life became a topsy-turvy struggle and our marriage was faltering under the strain.

Our daughter's weakened emotional condition, created by the sudden out-of-state move by her baby's father (he was to be the baby's caregiver) created the need for me to request an emergency leave of absence from my job as a special education aide. I would care for her baby while my daughter was student-teaching—student-teaching was the only portion of her schooling left to earn the elementary education degree she needed to secure her future. Though I had been a dedicated district employee for eleven years, the unpaid, short-term leave I requested was denied. Unfortunately, I was caught up in the poor timing of a new superintendent and new special education supervisor; neither knew me. They didn't realize that I had spent the last eleven years totally devoted to my special education students. Leaving a rewarding, stable job to care for my granddaughter would be a financial burden and a difficult choice, but my heart knew it was the only *right* choice.

From the time I was a young girl, my parents had instilled in me a love of nature, of all the best, beautiful, free things that life had to offer. Now, more than ever, I would need to draw on that love of nature; it would provide me with the strength needed to pull through the rough times. I began to take long walks with my granddaughter and I found that I would return home physically and spiritually renewed. Autumn was upon us; Alyssa would giggle with delight whenever I placed a leaf or a dried dandelion on the tray of her stroller.

As the trees became bare, I became aware of bird's nests that had been hidden in the dense summer foliage. "Alyssa, look—a little bird's nest," I would say. One of the most beautiful nests we found was a tiny, circular one created from bits of dried grasses. The weaving was tight, strong, and yet soft to the touch. Surely it would have rivaled one of Frank Lloyd Wright's creations. Some were crafted from feathers, dryer lint and bits of pet fur. Still other nests were masterpieces of corn silks, twine, strands of Easter grass and cellophane. How resourceful those little birds were! Each day, my eyes were drawn upward as I discovered more nests. Some were reinforced with mud, forming super strong foundations. Through wind, rain, thunder and lightning, they held together. I began to think about the birds—how simple, yet how hard their lives were. It occurred to me that no matter what obstacles were placed in their path, they managed to overcome, to survive. And faithfully, they started each new day with a song.

Those walks helped transform an extremely difficult, desperate time in my life to a more peaceful one. Through my observations of nature, I had faith that everything would work out and we would prevail. Like the birds and their nests, our family had a strong foundation. We were now living a more simple life, spending only what we needed to spend, and all the time becoming more resourceful. Courageously, the little birds of the air huddle close during stormy times, and the current turbulence seemed to be drawing our family closer together. And in the same way that the little birds started each day with a song, we began to listen to beautiful music more often. A sense of tranquility was settling over our home.

Time has a way of healing, of smoothing over the bumpy parts of our lives. Gradually we see things from a different perspective. One afternoon, while out walking with my granddaughter, I witnessed the most exceptional message of all from the birds. "Look at the geese, Alyssa," I said, as a flock of geese flew overhead in a perfect V formation. For some odd reason, one goose left the group and started to fly in an entirely different direction. The main flock completely changed its course and gradually picked up their wayward member. As I watched this simple, beautiful display, I couldn't help but think of my family. Our lives too, it seemed, had gone astray for a while. But through courage, inner strength and pure love, our family would change its course and triumph. I knew that all would be well.

Susan Siersma

LIFE LESSON #2:
RECOGNIZE YOUR STRENGTHS

The vast majority thinks that through criticism or judgment one can shame oneself into being different. But this rarely works. Most people don't respond well to disparagement; in fact, they usually become defensive and resistant. You're no different. In order to make the changes necessary to create the life you want, you have to shift your position from focusing on your flaws and shortcomings to recognizing your strengths, talents and positive qualities. You have to create a foundation of love and support.

Don't get us wrong, we're not suggesting that you become a Pollyanna, but that you maintain a balanced, compassionate view of yourself. Everything you've done, everyone you've loved, every mistake you've made, every obstacle you've overcome, is part of the woman you are today.

Questions Worth Asking

- What are three things I've accomplished in my life that I'm most proud of?
- What are five of my strengths, talents, and positive qualities? (Yes, you do have them. If you spend a little time, you'll find that there are far more than five.)
- How do I use my gifts and strengths in everyday life?
- Are there ways in which I could make better use of my resources?

> *That which will not kill you . . . will only make you stronger.*
>
> *Friedrich Nietzsche*

Change occurs most readily from a foundation of acceptance and support. A committed, nurturing relationship with yourself is essential. The only way you will create a life you love is with one caring, compassionate act at a time. You have to love and appreciate yourself into wholeness. You need to be there for yourself if you're going to change the things in your life that are robbing you of living your best life.

I acknowledge and accept myself for who I am.

☕ With a Little Help from a Stranger

*Until you make peace with who you are, you'll
never be content with what you have.*

DORIS MORTMAN

I met a friend of a friend when they included me in their lunch plans. My friend is a rare enough bird so I could have anticipated that her friends would rise, exponentially, on the scale of non-traditional species. No surprise, then, when I was led into a home eclectically decorated with exotic remnants of extraordinary places. Not a spoon collection or snow globe in this riverfront bungalow. How about a coconut shell, carved into a totem likeness of my hostess; "a gift from the shaman," she explained casually.

Over lunch I had to pretend perfect calm as I noted not one but four wasps buzzing at the overhead plant in her kitchen. "Oh, those are rescued. I had to save their hive and they live in here and on the patio. They won't hurt you."

And they didn't.

She supported herself as a freelance art photographer. Her work was tastefully exhibited in discreet clusters. Her name was something ethereal, full of A's and R's, requiring a leisurely roll about the tongue. She was one of the most genuine humans I had ever chanced to meet.

And so it was that in the presence of the free-range wasp colony, ice water with the freshest twist of lemon and a lunch of hummus on pita bread, this most unusual of creatures turned to me, full and attentive, sincere and with absolute meaning and said, "Tell me about you."

I like to think I'm articulate enough, having suffered enough showers and spousal work gatherings to know small talk with some flair, but nothing prepared me for "Tell me about you."

"Well, I. . . ."

She really wanted to know!

"I guess I'm . . ."

She was still paying attention. She wanted me to tell her about Me.

So, I suppose I stammered about being a nurse or a grandmother or winters in Minnesota. I'm not sure. I was quite unsure of my role in this question, and further, my role in my own world.

It was a take-home gift, that kind query. I don't think I was meant to answer it properly there, or ever, for her. If I'm not what I do, or a person in a relationship, or a resident of a particular place, but all that and none of that, then tell me about me.

If I could return to that luncheon table, wasps singing above (still safe in her presence, I'm sure), I would try to answer her. I might talk about the things I wish for and the things that make me unexpectedly happy, or the darkest thoughts I've ever had to sweep from my mind. I might tell her the things I pretend to be or to feel or to understand when I really don't believe a bit of it. How about when I should be sad but am really only angry, or when I seem red-hot angry but really feel ice-blue with fear? What if I told her all the things I wonder about and how little I know for sure?

So, on those days when uncertainty reigns supreme and I'm tempted to skitter off into a familiar pattern of internal chaos, I can take myself, for just a moment, back to that warm, blessed kitchen table in the house by the river and begin, "Let me tell you about Me."

I'm the one who needs to attend to the conversation that follows.

Beadrin Youngdahl

LIFE LESSON #3:
GET TO KNOW THE REAL YOU

At this point you might be asking yourself, what are they talking about? I know myself. After all, I'm with myself twenty-four hours a day, seven days a week. How much better can I know me? You spend so much of your time focused on your relationships with other people that you often neglect the most important relationship of all—the relationship with yourself.

Authentic
\∂-'thent-ik\ *worthy of acceptance or belief as conforming to fact or reality: syn. genuine, veritable, bona fide; being actually and precisely what is claimed.*

The majority of women are so caught up in their lives that they've forgotten who they truly are. When someone asks you to introduce yourself, do you respond by telling them what you do, where you live or who you know? Those are certainly important aspects of your life, but they aren't your whole life—or at least they shouldn't be.

Women are so identified with their roles as mother, wife, caretaker, daughter and sometimes career woman that they often lose track of themselves. Women forget who they are beyond these roles. They forget who they

wanted to be, what they dreamt of
becoming, what they love, what they
value. In effect, they've forgotten their
"sel

"sel

W
diffe
esse
part
ishe
evid

M
auth
stru
or t

[handwritten note covering text:]

Family
Friends
Belonging
Discovering / travel
Creativity

effort to sustain this image is both
draining and self-defeating, and it
requires too much energy to maintain.
It's time to step free of the scripted life
you've been living and search for who
you really are in the depth of your being. Peel away
everything that's not essential and discover your authentic identity. Reclaim the woman you truly are!

Remember what's most important in your life.
Remember your hopes and dreams. Discover or rediscover
your deepest yearnings. In order to do this, you need to

Questions Worth Asking

- How do the people in my life see me? What do they come to me for?

- What role do I play most often: care-taker, teacher, nur-turer, risk taker, rebel, diplomat, the responsible one?

- How has playing this role served me? Does it still serve me?

- How has playing this role blocked me from doing the things I truly enjoy?

embark on a psychological search-and-rescue mission to comb back through your life and recover your joy, wisdom, passion, enthusiasm, self-confidence, vitality—the threads of your true self that you lost along the way.

Creating a life you love requires courage, commitment and perseverance. All of which you have. The call now is for you to be authentically yourself.

I am reconnecting with my authentic self and reclaiming my true joys and passions.

☕ Follow Your Heart

I am an ocean person, though I have lived most of my life away from the sea I love so much. When I was forty-two, I had been longing for it for so many years, I began to feel my soul was dying.

I had been a single mother of four, it felt like, forever, since the youngest was an infant. I raised my children entirely on my own, through poverty and struggle, but with lots of laughter, kite-flying and hiking in the hills above our town—lots of grit and determination to do the best I could for these four people entrusted to my care. I was working at a job I hated, waiting for the older three to be finished with high school, feeling like I was marking time while the precious years flew by. I looked around me at the scenery of the Okanagan everyone else thought so beautiful. But for me it was the wrong scenery. Placid lake instead of frothing waves; brown hillsides instead of wild and verdant forest. I was in the wrong place and felt like I existed only to haul brown paper bags of groceries through the front door.

That birthday, my sister gave me a late autumn trip to see the gray whale migration outside of Tofino on the wild,

West Coast I longed for. Though I had never seen it, I just knew that there the waves would be wild and nature would be at its unfettered best, untamable by man.

It was as perfect an experience as it could possibly be: We were in a Zodiac, the ocean was serene, there were whales everywhere, the day was clear and sharply etched and, when we turned off the motor and drifted, we were on the same level as the whales. In fact, they were so unconcerned with our presence that one whooshed up close beside the boat, thrilling me to my toes. We passed by rocks covered with sea lions, who barked imperiously at our passage with a strange growly sound that delighted me; we sat beneath a huge eagle's nest and stared at the resident eagle, who stared diffidently back at us; little orange-beaked puffins bobbed serenely on neighboring waves; we investigated little forested inlets and found a waterfall. And to top it off, as we headed back to shore, sunset spread its palette of color before us. It was perfection. The guides who owned the boat were environmentalists; there was talk of saving this last precious ecosystem, this last stand of old growth. Everything I loved, longed for and believed in was here, and I wondered: *Why am I not here too?*

Time for one fast stop at the beach heading out and then the day was gone and I went back to my home in the Okanagan, to my hated job, and to a persistent depression as winter closed in. I wrote a letter, after a few weeks, telling the woman who had taken me to see the whales how lucky she was to be living her dream, and how long the West Coast had been my own dream. I had heard her mention she had never been able to find anyone who could take over her duties as well as she did them, so she could have more leisure time. I ventured in that letter to wonder if I might be that person, if there might be a place for me there.

There was no reply; the winter went on. The light in my eyes deadened, the walls closed in. I felt trapped—by the need to earn a living and support the kids, and by my aloneness (I had waited a long time for Mr. Right to come along and help me change my life; it was too hard and scary to do alone). I won recognition from an aware employer that my spirit was faltering; she encouraged me to take supervisory training and apply for the position of supervisor, to get me out of the job and shift work I hated and into another department—and management. I passed the training, won the position and for the first time was earning enough money to not have to worry on a daily basis about food and bills.

It was right then that the universe, in the form of a letter from Tofino, offered me the choice it has given me several times in my life: continued "security" (a huge issue for a single mother accustomed to poverty) or the life of my dreams: part-time work at six dollars an hour, but in Tofino where I most longed to be.

I wrestled a bit with the uncertainties, the hugeness of the choice, but there was little doubt. Though terrified and needing assurances that simply were not there, I knew this choice was between following my heart, or giving up my dream for financial reasons and staying where my spirit was dying. And I knew I couldn't live without a dream.

It is good I didn't know then what that choice entailed: the scarcity of rental housing of any kind, never mind affordable; the need to work two and three part-time, low-paying jobs at a time to survive; the exhaustion; the constant struggle; the first few years of continual moving.

What I did know is that, from the moment I set foot on the beach, that longing voice inside me was stilled. I was at home, the home of my spirit, the place in the world that was right for me. The night I rounded the corner at Long Beach in the rented moving truck, a gigantic orange ball of sun was dipping below the horizon, and the sky was a Gauguin canvas. Taking a moment from unloading boxes to stand on the front porch, I saw a whale in the bay—a whale in my front yard! The universe was saying: Hello! One dream, come true!

For ten years, I have walked ecstatically through some of the most spectacularly beautiful landscapes on the planet. Each and every day, joy and gratitude have resonated in my heart at the beauty upon which I feast. There is a fullness in me that means more now than any amount of money.

It took enormous courage, but I followed my heart and made my dream come true. I also learned that there is no security, other than what we carry within us. There is an inner voice that will guide us each and every step of the way when we slow down and choose to listen. When we heed this inner wisdom, our lives are enriched immensely. The road map for our journey can—indeed, must—be charted by our inner guide and the fulfillment of our dreams.

Sherry Baker

LIFE LESSON #4:
BE TRUE TO YOURSELF

At the end of a long life, the Hasidic rabbi Zusia announced before his death, "In the world to come no one will ask me why I was not Moses. I shall be asked, 'Why were you not Zusia?'"

Why indeed? Why isn't each woman the person she was intended to be? Why do women strive to be someone other than who they really are? It's time to stop trying to be who your parents expected you to become or what your spouse,

If we go down into ourselves we find that we possess exactly what we desire.

Simone Weil

partner or children want you to be. It's time to bring forth what is real and authentic about yourself.

As young women, many of you sought your identity and fulfillment in the outer world, and during the first half of your life that's appropriate. Yet as you attain success, you sense that there must be something more. With so much emphasis in this culture on achievement, it's easy to overlook the importance of your inner life.

One of the best ways to reconnect with your essential self is to listen to that still, small voice of your heart and above all, heed the wisdom of the philosopher, Diogenes: "Know thyself."

Shakespeare said, "To thine own self be true"; Plato advised, "The unexamined life is not worth living"; and Jesus advised his followers, "The Kingdom of God is within you." You must now make a choice—a choice of how you're going to live your life. Are you going to be dictated by the need to prove yourself and please other people or are you going to discover a deeper, truer sense of purpose?

Today I am bringing forth what is
real and true about myself.

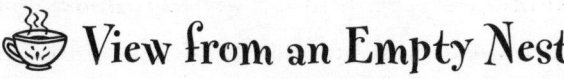 View from an Empty Nest

You are the hero of your own story.

MARY McCARTHY

Years ago when I first heard the term "empty nest," it sounded like a pleasant position to be in. I had three toddlers and the thought of waking up in the morning fully rested, instead of having my eyes pried open by tiny fingers, was quite attractive.

I correctly assumed that in an empty nest, I could wear clothes without spit-up stains, finish sentences when speaking to my husband, and carry a purse without squeak toys, or pacifiers, or cookie crumbs.

Oh, the beauty of dinnertime without spilled milk, a house without the background sounds of crying, walls without sticky fingerprints, and being able to sleep through an entire night. I could push a shopping cart that was filled with groceries instead of children!

However, when I reached that sought-after goal, it was rather a disappointment. Up close, the empty nest no longer looked quite as attractive. This was partly because the ensuing years had automatically solved many of the distasteful parts of motherhood. For some time, no one had been spitting up on me or crying to be fed in the middle of the night. Nobody needed to be bathed or dressed or have their shoes tied ten times a day. Just when the children became pleasant company, they moved out. Is there no justice?

I tried not to look into the three empty bedrooms as I passed by them. Even though the beds were all neatly made, the rooms lacked character. The one-eyed teddy bear was missing from his favorite spot on the floor. School books, papers, and cans of hair spray had all disappeared. The closet doors covered vacant areas that at one time had been stuffed beyond their limits.

When I finally crept out of my depression to take a peek around me, I noticed my dear husband, Jack, looking almost the same as when I had fallen wildly in love with him. Except for showing a bit of wear and tear, the years had been good to him. I fondly looked at the gray hairs at his temple, knowing exactly where they had come from. I caught myself grinning when I realized that the creases on his face were smile lines, not worry wrinkles.

As I sat gazing at him, I realized my nest was not empty after all. It still held the one special person I had chosen to share my life with. In the quiet of the empty nest, it might be easier for us to find each other. As I looked at him

I wondered if maybe, just maybe, we could rekindle the sparks we had originally ignited. And then, as if to answer my unspoken question, he looked up at me and winked.

June Cerza Kolf

LIFE LESSON #5:
DISCOVER WHERE YOU RESIDE IN THE STORY OF YOUR LIFE

Each of you has lived many lives. No, we're not talking about reincarnation. We're talking about the chapters in your life through which you've evolved—childhood, adolescence, young adulthood, marriage, motherhood, and for some, divorce or death ~~~~ very chapter you've experienced ~~~~ ~~more~~ importantly, you have devel ~~~~ and preferences. It's time to bec ~~~~ gate your own life.

marriage – Andy
motherhood – Australia

Each of your experience ~~~~ lues upon which you've built your life, the things you've loved, the dreams you've fulfilled, the moments of satisfaction you've cherished. These hints, when remembered, will reveal what is needed to create a more genuinely fulfilling life. Your past reminds you of challenges you've endured, strengths you've accumulated, and the wisdom you've extracted from your experiences. After all, there's a direct connection between where you've been and where you're going. This awareness of your past and the choices you've made is the first step in creating your best life.

As I look back over my life, I appreciate where I've been and how far I've come.

Basic Tool: Your Journal

A journal is an invaluable tool. It's a place where you can begin a dialogue with yourself. It's a way for you to get to know yourself more intimately, to become your own confidante. Your journal will help you to become more introspective and self-reflective.

Make an agreement with yourself to keep your journal private, that you're not going to show it to anyone and that it's a safe place in which you can explore your thoughts, feelings, hopes, fears, dreams—anything that wants to be expressed. The key to using a journal is that you allow yourself to express whatever comes up with no censoring and no judging. Just allow a free flow of expression.

We'd like you to do what we call a Life Review. This exercise will help you recognize who you are and the path that has led you to where you are today. Although your life must be lived by moving forward, it is best understood by recognizing what you have already lived through and how far you've come. Just as your fingerprints identify your unique physical makeup, your "life choices" will reveal the person who did all the living—your self.

You need only claim the events of your life to make yourself yours. When you truly possess all you have been and done, which may take some time, you are fierce with reality.

Florida Scott Maxwell

People who've had near-death experiences often report engaging in a life review. This process is conducted in an atmosphere of unconditional compassion and understanding. We'd like to recommend that you embrace a similar attitude as you embark on this exercise.

A good way to get started with your Life Review is to divide your life into decades. Pull out your old photo albums and look at pictures of yourself during the different periods of your life. Put on some music from that time. Trace your life back to when you were in middle school, high school, the decade between eighteen and twenty-eight, from twenty-eight to thirty-eight, and so on. Discover what memories are kindled as you renew your acquaintance with the woman you were during each of these decades.

Answer the questions below.

[...] of weeks, spend fifteen min-
u[...] Life Review. Go decade by
d[...] begin by asking yourself the fol-
l[...]

> What three people influenced me most during this period of my life?
>
> What one event had a major impact on my life?
>
> How does that event affect my life today?
>
> What challenges did I overcome?
>
> What successes did I accomplish?
>
> What gave me the greatest sense of satisfaction or pride?
>
> Were there any compromises I made? What impact do they have on my current life? Is there anything I sacrificed that I'd now like to reclaim?
>
> What did I like to do?
>
> Who were my friends?

Through this Life Review, you'll not only gain insights into yourself, but you'll become more comfortable in your own skin. You'll have a greater appreciation of all that you've been through, your major accomplishments, and your major decisions and the roads not taken. As you do this, you can't help but have a renewed appreciation of your worth. No matter what improvements you may want to make, your life already *is* a success.

☕ PTA Mom

Elementary school brought two things: lice and the PTA. Both landed squarely in my lap and I'm not sure which was worse. Lice, beastly little vermin that they are, eventually went away. Of course, it took two months and almost two hundred dollars worth of shampoos and sprays for the whole family—not to mention the additional laundry. But no matter what I scrub, I just can't get rid of the PTA.

I should explain that part of the problem is that I have a genetic disorder called "martyr's syndrome." My mother has it too. What it does is cause us to jump up and run around screaming "I can do it! Pick me! Pick me!" any time *anyone*, and I do mean anyone, mentions that they might need help with something. It doesn't matter what it is. We volunteer. Need someone to pick up your kids even though it's painfully inconvenient? I'll do it. Want your driveway stenciled in cute little bunnies? No problem. Need a position filled for the PTA? Well, I'm your gal.

Certifiably nuts is what I am.

The first year was a cakewalk. I was a room mother. I don't know who I impressed but this year I'm not only a room mother—head room mother to boot—but also on the Carnival Committee, the Committees Committee and Youth Protection Chairman, the latter being my formal title. A more accurate description would be Chief Patsy.

My husband often tells me he is under grave duress during the day, but has he ever had to put on a six-foot giant bug costume and entertain six hundred squealing kids ages four to ten?

Any mother willing to cram her ample body into head to toe yellow tights and don a Louie the Lightning Bug outfit deserves the Mother of the Year award. And I'm not saying that because I did it. No, I'm saying it because a total stranger had to pry me out of the blasted thing. Getting in is easy; getting out is a different story—just like the PTA.

It's work—hard, thankless work. Relax is not in the vocabulary of a PTA mom. But boy, oh boy, volunteer is. The other day I was trying unsuccessfully to weasel a neighbor, a mom with three kids, into volunteering for the school carnival. Her excuse for not helping out at the carnival was, "I like to keep my weekends free."

Free? With three kids?

I go to the bathroom with two kids and the dog staring at me. I take a shower with a door that mysteriously swings open every two seconds because my toddler wants in or my husband can't find the kitchen. Nothing breaks or disappears until I get in the bathroom.

My only comfort is knowing that I am not alone. The mommas I pass in the school's halls every day have the same glassy-eyed look I do. We catch ourselves frantically patting our clothing to make sure it's on right-side out before we enter the school. Forget matching clothing. This is elementary school. Most of the kids dress themselves. Do you think the teachers will notice one more set of clashing colors? I've seen these kids. It's a wonder the teachers aren't colorblind out of self-preservation.

It's a good thing they don't expect us to look like June Cleaver. June Cleaver never had to chase a greased naked little boy who anointed himself and the cat with a super-sized bottle of baby oil, or scrape peanut butter off the toilet seat. Who has time for makeup and pearls? I'm lucky to brush my hair. The teachers, bless their hearts, don't care if we're naked. They're so glad to see parents who care enough to show up and do *something*.

Which is why the PTA gets under your skin. Thankless, yes. More work than you thought, yes. Aggravating and annoying, yes, yes. But when I peeled out of that god-awful bug getup, all sweaty and unappealing, my daughter hugged me and said, "You were great! You're the best mom ever!"

That's why, no matter how much it makes me itch, I just can't shake the PTA. And maybe, just *maybe*, I love it.

K. K. Choate

Life Lesson #6:
Recognize What's Important

One of the cornerstones of living a high quality life is to know what you value—what's most meaningful in your life. Yet when your life is all about completing the millions of tasks on your "to do" list, it's easy to lose perspective. You lose your ability to discern what's important from what's not because everything feels equally urgent, equally critical.

No matter how frantic life gets, the truly successful people are able to rise above the pandemonium and maintain their perspective. They can do this because they know what's important. Their values are their compass—they keep them on course regardless of the confusion of life. These people maintain a vision of what truly matters, what their life is about and what they want it to be.

Think about the qualities and attributes that you consider essential to living your best life. These are the values you use to define yourself. For example, your

Questions Worth Asking

- What are my top 10 core values and principles?
- What are five qualities I'd like to be remembered for?
- What have I found myself saying to the world over and over throughout my life?

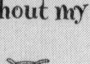

list could include such attributes as: Integrity, honesty, play-fulness, understanding, trustworthiness, responsibility, truth, creativity, adventurousness. Remember these are just a few suggestions. There are many more possibilities. Come up with a list that reflects *your* core values—not what you think you should value, but what you feel is truly important to you.

By clarifying your values you can adjust your life so that you invest your time and energy in those things you hold sacred. Asking yourself, "What do I value? What's most important to me? What do I really want?" will not only help you understand yourself on a deeper level, but ultimately refocus your life around what's truly meaningful. It's actually less important to understand the meaning of life than it is to under-stand the meaning of *your* life.

Now that you have a clearer picture of what you consider important, ask yourself: What do I need to change in order to have my values expressed more visibly in my everyday life? Is there anything I need to add to my life? Are there activities or commitments I need to eliminate?

> ### Food for Thought
>
> Ask yourself every day, Is this what I want to be doing? If the answer is "no," you can, day-by-day, begin to alter your course. Changing course is a process—it happens slowly, incrementally. But if you are persistent you will end up where you want to be.
>
>

We offer you this challenge—remain focused on who you truly are, what you believe in, and what you love. As you do, you will begin to create a life in which your outer life matches your more deeply held values and beliefs. This feeling of being "all of a piece" is an Essential Ingredient in living the life you were meant to live.

I am true to my deeply held values and my life reflects what is most meaningful to me.

The Finishing Touch

WRITE A LETTER TO YOURSELF

It's time to sit right down and write yourself a letter. Just as Deborah Shouse did in the story "The Love Letter," remember what you love, cherish, appreciate and even admire about yourself. Sure, it's going to feel awkward at first, but the truth is that only to the extent that you love and value yourself are you able to love and support others.

Make an agreement with yourself to allow whatever you are feeling to flow onto your paper. Don't censor yourself, and above all, don't judge what it is you have to say. Simply write a letter to a trusted friend and confidant, sharing whatever is in your heart. If there are any questions or decisions you are considering, use this opportunity to ask yourself for guidance. You may want to ask questions such as:

What's in my best interest?

What do I need to do to take better care of myself?

Are there any insights that can help me grow as a person or make my life more balanced?

What do I love, cherish and admire about myself?

Once you've finished, be sure to save your letter for those times when you need a pick-me-up or a pep talk.

TAKE CHARGE OF YOUR LIFE

*How we spend our days is, of course,
how we spend our lives.*

Annie Dillard

☕ Taking the Leap

Everything's in the mind.
That's where it all starts. Knowing what
you want is the first step towards getting it.

MAE WEST

One winter morning, the love of my life died from the love of his life, 120-proof vodka. We'd been apart a long time, yet when I cleaned his apartment with my stepdaughters, we found an unfinished letter to me in his typewriter. "Don't be afraid," it read. "You are a survivor."

Yes, I thought, *but is surviving all I want out of life? Who did I used to be, anyway? What happened to the poet in me?*

I visited a career counselor several times. He said the tests he administered showed I scored highest in writing and the creative arts. But I was winning awards at my civil service job, I told him, and I was up for another raise. It would be crazy to leave at forty, to start all over again as a novice writer. He reluctantly agreed. "But how about seeing what you can do after work hours," the counselor suggested. "See if you can find more ways to express yourself."

I kept on plodding to my government job, day after day, but I also worked on finding outlets for my hobbies. My church choir was glad to have me join. I was so happy at choir practice, the quiet alto beside me confessed one day that she envied me. "You're such a free spirit," she said. I also began to sell occasional pieces of my hand-thrown pottery. "It must be wonderful to have that talent," someone remarked. Best yet, I started writing feature articles for local publications. "Gee," a friend said, "I wish I had the courage to send in something I've written."

Free spirit? Talent? Courage? What a fraud I was! If I really had courage, I told myself, I'd take that step into the abyss. Get out of a job that was killing my soul and devote myself full-time to anything related to writing. But I feared what might be waiting for me outside: growing poor, being thought silly and irresponsible. Failing.

It was a couple of weeks before Christmas the following year. Lights were strung all over town; carols echoed from the street-lamp speakers. But I wasn't into the holidays. I hid in bed a lot, cursing my so-called talents, feeling stuck. Why couldn't I simply tend to my present job, collect my pay, watch TV, and stop the adolescent angst over my life's meaning and goals? My job was interfering with my real work in life, and I knew it.

That night my bedside phone rang; it was a friend from my church choir. "I have very sad news," she told me. Our alto friend, the one who envied me, had killed herself. At her memorial service, while everyone spoke so lovingly of my friend, I remembered what she had said to me: "You're so free . . . outrageous . . . courageous."

I knew at that moment that if I didn't follow my own calling, I might someday follow her path. For days the old maxims kept coming to mind: Know thyself. Be true to yourself. Have the courage of your convictions.

Do or die.

I examined my lifestyle. What were my priorities? Staying alive, not just in body, but also in spirit. I made plans. I'd have to stretch my abilities and skills, hustle for a living as never before. But I decided within those few days to make my friend's death have meaning for me; I'd make what she saw in me the truth.

As I worked out my notice, excitement and fear became my midnight playmates.

The "what-ifs" raged. But I continued to clear my office. Down came all that said I'd been there for more than ten years, including my framed Kierkegaard quote: "Life can only be understood backwards, but it must be lived forwards." Now I finally understood the quote.

It's been many years since I declared my independence. I've learned that working for myself means long hours, and that writing alone doesn't pay my bills. But I've never looked back. The years since I stepped off into my own abyss have flown. Most mornings, I wake excited about my work, whether it's writing one of my columns, meeting article deadlines, teaching college writing or coaching another writer. I don't succeed at everything I try. Sometimes I fall on my face, but it's not from standing still.

Erma Bombeck once wrote a column that felt like a personal letter to me. She said, "I always had a dream that when I am asked to give an accounting of my life to a higher court, it will go thusly. 'So, empty your pockets. What have you got left of your life? Any dreams that were unfulfilled? Any unusual talent that we gave you when you were born that you still have left?'

"And I will answer," Bombeck continued, "'I've nothing to return. I spent everything you gave me. I'm as naked as the day I was born.'"

Me, too, I want to tell Bombeck. Me, too.

K. K. Wilder

*Interior Design /
Styling
Decorating mood boards*

LIFE LESSON #1:
EVALUATE YOUR PRIORITIES

The French philosopher René Descartes said, "I think, therefore, I am." The modern-day version has become "I do, therefore, I am." So many women live by the mantras "I have to keep up," "I am what I do," "I have to push myself," "I have to prove my worth," "I have to keep going." While many of you thought that you left peer pressure back in the halls of high school, it's still very much in operation in your adult lives.

Many women have one clear priority: get through the day. Sure, no one would deny the importance of that, but it's simply not enough. You go through life on autopilot. You rarely stop long enough to consider how you spend your time and energy. Yet, without determining whether your priorities match your reality and your values, you will continually be out of synch with yourself.

Living a priority-centered life means balancing responsibility to others with responsibility to oneself, obligations with enjoyment, work with play, activity with rest. It means finding a natural rhythm to your day-to-day life that will support an atmosphere of fulfillment. It means getting your priorities straight.

Reach high, for stars lie hidden in your soul. Dream deep, for every dream preceded the goal.

Pamela Vaull Starr

Think of a typical day and a typical week. Think about how you spend your time. Ask yourself, how much time do I devote to my family? What about health and fitness? Religion or spiritual practice? Work? Personal interests and hobbies? Social time? Finances? Friendships? The categories you choose may look somewhat different from these, so feel free to customize them to reflect your life. Make a list in order of what gets the most to the least amount of your time. How you spend your time will reveal your priorities.

You may be surprised to discover that there's a discrepancy be~~tween~~ thought your priorities ~~are and where~~ they actually are. It's ti~~me to get honest~~ with yourself and see w~~hat your life is~~ telling you. Is your life ~~balanced? Are~~ you overextended in one area? Is there an~~ area you're~~ neglecting? What percentage of your tim~~e is spent~~ caring for others? What percentage is s~~pent nurturing~~ yourself and doing things you love? Are you in synch with your core values? Are there any adjustments you need to make so that your life more closely reflects these values?

[handwritten list:] list — family — fitness — religion — work — hobbies — social — finances — friendships

One of the greatest challenges women face is balancing the wishes and expectations of other people (especially your family) with your *own* needs and desires. Hold your priorities sacred. Invest your time and energy in what you value. Commit yourself to making time for what's important every single day.

I am getting my priorities straight.
My life reflects my deepest held values and beliefs.

☕ Communing with Nature

Almost every morning before I start my day, I make my way to this little park. Very seldom do I see anyone else there. It seems that everyone else is too busy running here and there to stop to admire God's beautiful creation.

It was quiet at the little pond that morning. The water was still. The leaves on the trees were not shivering like usual. The silence was broken by the ringing of my cellular phone. The noise startled me. I jumped and grabbed the telephone wondering who would be calling me that early.

"Hi, Mama," my son, Chad, said. "What are you doing?"

"I'm sitting at a little pond across town," I answered.

"You're doing what?" he inquired.

"I'm spending some quiet time at this perfect little place," I explained. "I come here almost every morning. It helps me get my day started on the right track."

"You're sitting at a pond communing with nature, while I'm stuck in Atlanta traffic," Chad laughed. "It must be nice."

"It is very nice," I admitted. "You should try it some time."

Chad and I talked until the traffic resumed on his end.

We offered our loving farewells and hung up.

My mind took me to a place where I had lived several years earlier. I was one of those people living every minute of each day in a rat race. I didn't take the time to commune with nature, spend quiet time with God, or take the time to get in touch with my feelings. I thought I was happy driving in the fast lane of life.

When I think back I realize that I had been afraid of being alone. I could put on a good show before everyone else, but if I got quiet I was forced to be honest with myself. I wasn't doing the things that I knew deep in my heart I was supposed to be doing. God had called me to minister to others through writing and public speaking, but I had ignored His call. I justified my actions by telling myself that I had to make a living. I was exactly like everybody else in this world—struggling to make ends meet, while not considering the real reason for my existence.

I was afraid to slow down. *If I miss a day at work, I will get too far behind,* I reasoned. Therefore, I worked even when I was sick. I pushed myself to the limit so many times. I wondered who I was trying to impress. Was it my boss or coworkers? I decided that it was probably me that I was trying to impress. I had to feel worthy. I wanted to feel like a dedicated and hard-working employee. But in the meantime, I denied myself the privilege of really living my life to its fullest.

I took a few more minutes to pray. A few birds landed in the tree beside me. I smiled as I listened to the songs they were singing. A squirrel scampered by, but not without stopping to gaze at me. I glanced at my watch and knew that my quiet time was over. It was time to start my day.

I stood before a group of ladies at a speaking engagement. "Today is the first day of the rest of your lives," I announced. "Where will you go from here?" I shared the story about the pond, my son's remark, and the emotions I felt that morning while communing with nature and God.

I encouraged the ladies to slow down, serve God each and every day, and to take some time to pray. The meeting concluded about an hour later, and I returned to my car. I felt good. I was no longer afraid to leave my comfort zone for God's sake. I was thankful that I gave up the fast lane of life. I was excited to be doing the things that God created me to do.

I drove back to the pond before I returned home from my engagement. The wind had picked up. I watched as the ripples in the once still water traveled to the shore. I realized that the words I share at my speaking engagements can be compared to the ripples in the water. By spreading the good news to others, they can find the peace and joy that only God and nature can give.

Nancy B. Gibbs

LIFE LESSON #2: REORIENT YOUR LIFE

Stop and consider for a moment what would happen if you took the next available exit on the freeway of your life, pulled onto a quiet country lane, slowed down and reflected. What would happen if you asked yourself, Am I doing too much? Am I doing enough? Am I living the life I want to live? As you ponder these questions you may discover that you want to make some changes. You may find that you need to reassess your priorities based on what you've determined is most meaningful in your life. You may decide that you need more balance, more time for yourself. You may realize that you have to take greater charge of where you invest your time and energy.

In the last section, you clarified your priorities. Now it's time to think about reorienting your life to reflect what's most important to you now. But remember, your priorities are not written in stone. They need to be adaptable and to change as you do.

The purpose of life, after all, is to live it, to taste experience to the utmost, to reach out eagerly and without fear for newer and richer experience.

Eleanor Roosevelt

If you're like most people, you probably spend most of your time trying to keep up with your "to do" list before you

rself to get to the good stuff. All
you put your own needs on the
have time" list rather than on
do" list. These kinds of choices
g you away from the life you

Rather than saying "I don't have time to exercise or play with my kids or take a piano lesson," take responsibility for your decisions. Say, "I could do what I want if I tried this a different way," or "Why is this my top priority?" How you spend your time is *your* choice. It's all too easy to blame other people, but when you take full responsibility for your time, you have the power to make changes. You *do* have time for what's important.

Questions Worth Asking

- Where will I be in 10 years if I continue on the path I'm on today?

- Is it where I want to be? If not, what can I do to start making a change today?

- What actions can I take to bring greater balance into my life?

- When I'm 80, what will I regret having done or not done?

Basic Tool: Priorities List

Make a list of the five things you most want in your life in order of importance. For example, your priorities might be:

1. exercising
2. spending time with your children
3. getting your finances in shape
4. your spiritual life
5. friends

Next to each activity, list the amount of time you currently devote to that item in the course of a typical week. How does your present life match the life you want to be living? Are there any adjustments that need to be made?

Now that you know what's important to you, use this information as a guide when making choices. Before you agree to something, ask yourself, is this in alignment with my priorities? Will this activity or commitment enhance my life or detract from creating the life I want?

I am reorienting my life around what is most important to me.

☕ The Art of Saying "No"

The downside of the friendship didn't present itself right away. She was one of the first people to welcome my family to our new community five years earlier. An outgoing woman with children the same ages as mine, she volunteered countless hours at our kids' grade school. One day you could find her applying ice packs in the health room, the next straightening collars for school pictures. And that was when she wasn't putting together the school directory or stenciling the lunchroom.

My kids liked her son and daughter, and frankly, I did, too. They were so well-mannered, addressing me as "Mrs. McQuestion" and asking permission before using my bathroom. Their mother was a great conversationalist who told interesting stories about the people and history of our small town.

It started out innocently enough. My new friend would call to chat and somewhere in the conversation she'd ask me to help with the book fair or baseball registration. If I hesitated, she'd tell me how lucky I was to work from home and how much helping would benefit my kids. I always caved. A pattern developed; she took on too many volunteer activities and increasingly counted on me to pick up the slack.

Over time I realized that I was getting roped into doing far more than I wanted. I loved the flexibility of working from home, but more and more I saw it as a disadvantage. I dreaded the sound of her voice on the phone, knowing that I was about to get shanghaied into service.

Once after listening to me grumble, my husband grinned and said, "You're her toady."

"I am not." I was indignant. Then I looked up "toady" in the dictionary, and like the old joke, saw my photo next to the definition. Thinking back, I had to admit to a lifelong tradition of people pleasing—doing favors only because I wanted to be liked. I had a history of handling unwanted requests with lame excuses, hoping my reluctance would speak for itself. My last resort was to say I didn't want to (work the refreshment booth, unload the cookie truck, etc.), but would if they really couldn't find anyone else. Guess what? They never found anyone else. I thought it was my destiny to be tromped upon.

This was one character trait I couldn't blame on my mother. The family joke was that Mom didn't need assertiveness training—she could teach the course. When I was growing up, she got the same types of phone calls— the church needed help with the craft fair, neighbors needed a babysitter, the elementary school wanted cookies for the bake sale. Mom listened politely. If she wanted to do it, she did. If not, she turned them down, hung up the phone and never thought about it again. She made it look easy.

Not that she didn't do her share. Mom raised four daughters, taught grade school for more than twenty years and still managed to be, at one time or another, a Brownie leader, Sunday school teacher and room mom. But she did it on her terms.

Mom had a standard line she used to politely decline requests. "That won't work out for me," she'd say. If the caller persisted she repeated the line, "It just won't work out for me." My sisters and I used to laugh at the vagueness of the phrase, but now I understand the sheer genius of it. It says nothing but conveys everything. As an added bonus, it leaves nothing open to argument. If it won't work out for you that's pretty much the end of it. What more is there to say?

"I don't owe them an explanation," Mom would say. "I just don't want to do it." In Mom's world anyone was free to ask and she was just as free to say no.

Some time after my husband called me a toady and I reached my fortieth birthday, I hit a turning point and developed a backbone.

My friend called after that to ask if I'd help with a pizza sale. The timing was bad; I was backlogged with work and other projects at home. Luckily I had Mom's key phrase memorized. "Sorry, it just won't work out for me," I told her. Amazingly, she didn't get mad and found someone else to help. The event ran smoothly without me.

Apparently I had a choice in the matter all along. Which reminds me of another saying my mother (now happily retired and doing exactly as she pleases) is fond of: Nobody can take advantage of you unless you let them.

If only I had listened to her long ago.

Karen McQuestion

Life Lesson #3:
Set Limits

One of the cornerstones for creating a life you love is setting limits. However, before you can set limits with other people, you have to define your boundaries for yourself. This requires that you know what you need, how you feel and what is and isn't acceptable to you. That's a tall order, especially for women, considering that in our culture women are conditioned to be selfless.

Think wrongly, if you please, but in all cases think for yourself.

Doris Lessing

It's time to start to set limits. But first you have to know your bottom line. How do you determine this? The answer is surprisingly simple: Your feelings—especially feelings of anger, frustration and resentment—are the messengers that will bring you this valuable information.

Anger often signals that you aren't getting your needs met, or that you're overextended. Your feelings of frustration and resentment, which are anger's first cousins, let you know that you've compromised or sacrificed too much of yourself. These feelings often help you to define what it is you want and need for yourself and your life. When paid attention to, your anger can motivate and mobilize you to take action, to speak out on your own behalf and to set clear boundaries. If you're going to live a high-quality life, you have to awaken a healthy self-protectiveness and find a balance between the needs of others and your own.

One of the obstacles you may run into, especially as a woman, is that the people closest to you often don't want you to change. They want everything to remain the same. Your spouse, boyfriend, children, parents and friends aren't going to want you to set limits, and they certainly are not going to help you to do it. There is a certain amount of comfort in the familiar. Most people resist

Questions Worth Asking

- What am I doing in my day-to-day life that I wish I wasn't?
- What am I currently doing that is absolutely right for me?

change, but the short-term discomfort that establishing new boundaries may create is well worth the effort.

The people closest to you may initially resist, but once they see that you're committed to taking care of yourself, they will probably accept your decisions. In time, they may even support you. Why? Because when you set and maintain your boundaries, you'll be happier, healthier and more fun to be around.

Long-term change requires looking honestly at our lives and realizing that it's nice to be needed but not at the expense of our health, our happiness, and our sanity.

Ellen Sue Stern

Keep in mind that your boundaries aren't set in stone. You can change them as needed. However, when you set limits, you will reduce the stress in your life and carve out more time to have more of what you want.

The next time someone asks you to do something, determine what your limits are before responding. Ask yourself, What can I reasonably and joyfully do? What am I willing to do? And what do I want to do? These three questions will help you to establish boundaries before you reach the point of no return. For example, a coworker regularly asks you to cover for her so she can leave work early. You've been feeling irritated about this for sometime, but have agreed. The next time she asks, before you automatically respond, "Sure, no problem," remember, no more Ms. Nice Girl and say, "Sorry, but that's just not going to work for me." A limit has been set.

We're not suggesting that you turn into Attila the Hun and run over other people, but rather that you define what's right for you. You don't need to become shrill and strident to set firm boundaries. You simply need to be clear about what you will and won't tolerate, and make a commitment to stand your ground.

I am setting limits — and I am
comfortable with my decisions.

☕ Enjoying the Moment

There was a day a few months ago when some city workers came into our subdivision to repair the street. It was a warm day and my children had been outside playing all morning. As I was making beds, picking up toys, sorting dirty laundry and doing my other "mom" chores, I listened to the grind and scrape of the diesel machines working in front of my home.

Nearing lunchtime, I went to call my six children in. They weren't in the backyard playing on all the gym equipment we had purchased for their entertainment. They weren't in the side yard playing kickball or soccer. They were in the front yard with awed expressions on their faces watching the machines on the street dig and dump and fill.

I watched them for awhile—my grubby little throng— amazed they could stand so still for longer than a minute, but unlike them, I soon became bored and called them in. I could see they were reluctant to come inside.

"We was watching the tractors!" my three-year-old exclaimed, pointing as if I hadn't seen the enormous machines.

"Why?" I asked.

They all traded glances and shrugged their shoulders, and my nine-year-old answered for them all, "Because they're neat."

Later I thought about how enthralled they were with those big machines, as so many children are, and I myself had been when I was young. It made me sad to think that I have become so busy trying to keep up with everyday life that I've forgotten how to enjoy the everyday things. That while we as adults are so busy chasing the almighty dollar, we've forgotten that the simple pleasures we enjoyed as children are free, right in our own backyards, there for the taking.

One lazy afternoon while watching my children play, I started thinking about how differently the world looks through the eyes of an adult with so many responsibilities. All at once I realized that while I was trying to raise them to be perfect mini-adults who would then become perfect full-grown adults, my oldest child at eleven was essentially still that—a child! I felt my stomach drop as I recalled reprimanding them over and over about this and that and giving lectures on appropriate behavior. I cringed inwardly as I realized with clarity that I've essentially been telling them that it's wrong to behave as the children they are.

My five-year-old chose that moment to look over and give me a wave. She yelled, "Mom, watch!" and jumped off the swing seat in mid-swing and flew through the air. I held my breath until she landed in the sandbox without a major injury.

My first response was to let loose a barrage of admonishments about how she could have broken a leg or landed on one of her younger sisters, but just as I started to yell, I shocked myself by responding with, "Wow!" And I gave her a thumbs-up.

Suddenly I felt a pang of longing for the days of my own youth. The days when I, too, could romp and play without a care for cost- of-living increases and budgets and mortgages. The days when all that seemed to matter was that day, that moment.

Remembering the day with the machines working in the street, I walked across the yard to my children and asked if I, too, could join in the fun. For a moment, six pairs of eyes just stared at me in astonishment. Even though I spend all day—every day—with them, it had been a long time since I'd taken off my "Mom" hat and just enjoyed the day—the moment—as if it would last forever.

I let my children re-teach me that afternoon, for I'd forgotten that a whole world of fun could exist in a child's backyard. I'd forgotten how much fun it is to squish and squeeze fresh mud into patties and lay them on rocks to dry in the sun. Or how plucking the stem from a honeysuckle will reward you with a single sweet drop of "honey." Or how forbidden it feels to make a mud puddle with the garden hose and stomp in it just for the sheer fun of getting dirty. And how thrilling it is to climb just *one* branch higher in a tree and then from your perch in the sky, gaze over your tiny kingdom through innocent eyes and yell, "I'm the king of the world!"

I'd forgotten how your stomach does that flip-flop tickle when you swing so high that the seat practically falls out of the sky and at the last moment catches, pulling you back to do it again. Or how relaxing it is to lie on your back in the grass watching the dandelion fluff float by on a lazy summer breeze. Or how, when you use your imagination, the clouds can really look like bunnies and horses. And I'd forgotten what it was like to be dirty and sweaty and itchy and not even care, because there was still an hour to play before dinner.

There was once a time when a day seemed to last forever and yet now I feel there aren't enough hours in a day to do all that needs to be done. I now know that the days slip by all too quickly and so does a child's youth. Once it is gone, it can never be reclaimed no matter how badly we wish for it.

As for myself, I can only hope to capture a few stolen moments from my children's youth to remind me how precious these carefree days are for them. And I try not to question why they will go through the trouble to rake all the leaves in the yard into a big pile just to run and jump and stomp and kick them all over the yard again. Instead, I go outside and join them. Enjoy the moment with them. Because even though they don't, I know the moment won't last forever.

Stacey Granger

LIFE LESSON #4:
DEFLATE SUPER WOMAN

Most women have perfected the art of people pleasing. They have become so expert at thinking about everyone else that they've become a shadow of the women they were meant to be. They're afraid that if they set limits they'll be branded with the scarlet "S" for selfish.

When you bring yourself back into the equation, it often feels like you're breaking an unwritten law—women must always put other people's needs before their own; women must make sure that everyone is taken care of; women must never disappoint or cause anyone pain. Are these beliefs at the core of how you live your life? They are for many women. Trying to live up to these standards is not only impossible, it condemns you to what we call the Super Woman Syndrome.

You all know Super Woman. She's the woman who thinks

she can do everything. She's the woman who pretends to be all things to all people. But if we tear down the Super Woman façade we find a wrung-out, exhausted woman who couldn't say "no" if her life depended on it. She's continually overwhelmed and overextended, yet she can't stop filling her calendar with volunteer opportunities, lunch dates, business meetings, social engagements and after-school activities for her equally weary children. She rescues stray animals, always has someone staying at her house, and is constantly helping those in need.

Food for Thought

- Take a moment and ask yourself: What would I secretly like to do if I stopped considering other people's expectations and opinions? Why aren't I doing it?
- Who am I trying to please? What price am I paying?

Just ask and her automatic reaction is, "Yes, sure, I'll be glad to do it." She spreads herself so thin that she barely exists except for other people.

Truth be told, Super Woman is pretty miserable and in desperate need of some time off. If you resemble this description, *even vaguely,* it's time to reevaluate your life and your automatic responses. It's time to readjust your internal image and admit that you're simply an ordinary woman with needs of your own. This is a radical shift, but one that is essential.

Even if you've hung up your Super Woman cape (or perhaps have never donned it), it often remains a struggle to make your limits known. But take heart, over time it will get easier; in fact, it will eventually become second nature.

I am learning to be realistic
with my expectations.

☕ A Higher Education

Sometime in your life you will go on a journey.
It will be the longest journey you have ever taken.
It is the journey to find yourself.

KATHERINE SHARP

The excitement of her first school bus ride was written across her face with a wide six-year-old missing-tooth grin and dazzling eyes. "Bye, Mom!" she yelled as she scurried across the highway as the red-flashing lights of the bus shielded her from oncoming traffic. I raised my hand in a wave and choked out the words, "Have a good day, sweetheart," as a tiny tear rolled down my cheek. And in one grinding gear sound, the big yellow bus chugged forward. I could see my baby waving furiously with her blonde curls bouncing. I took a deep breath. My anxiousness about sending my youngest child off to school passed as quickly as the bus drove out of sight. It was replaced by my own nauseating anticipation—this was my first day of school, too.

Camouflaged in jeans and T-shirt with a new canvas pack strapped to my back, I headed my minivan in the opposite direction to begin my first day at the university. Oh, I had plenty of doubts: Was I too old? Would I fit in? Would the younger students think I was crazy? Could I really do this? After all, it had been almost twenty years since I had read a text book, taken class notes and written essays. But I needed to go.

I had always wondered what it would have been like to go to college. As the oldest girl in my blue-collar family, it wasn't considered important for me to get a degree. In my mother's eyes, the only girls who went to college graduated with an Mrs. Degree; and besides, it was more important to send my brother who was three years younger because he would have to support a family some day. There just wasn't enough money for both of us to go. So I went to work in an office after graduation.

For some strange reason, there was a fire in my gut that I'd never experienced before. Maybe it had something to do with my best friend dying from breast cancer, which made me take a good look at my life. And when I did, I realized that my own life hadn't even started yet. I had gone from being somebody's daughter to somebody's wife to somebody's mother—but had never become *somebody* myself.

When I told my family that I wanted to go to college, I faced opposition on every front. My mother couldn't understand why I wanted to go, because in her eyes, I had everything—two beautiful children, a four-bedroom home in the country, a new car and a husband who made enough money so I didn't have to work. What more could I possibly want? Then there was my husband, who fought the very idea that I would want to go to school; after all, when would I have time to make the meals, clean the house, do the laundry and run the children to scouts and dance class? And to discourage me further, he vowed that he wouldn't give me one penny to finance this ridiculous dream. The only people who supported me were my little girls, and they really didn't understand how much their lives were going to change because of my dream. In a few months, they would grumble because they would have to put their own clothes in their dressers and take turns doing the dishes at night. But, on that first day of school, none of the opposition mattered.

Driving those five miles to the university turned out to be one of the most important moments in my life. In fact, it was a turning point. The lesson that began on that balmy September day would enrich my life forever because I learned that facing fear is worth the risk. That change is good. That growth is stimulating. That accepting challenges and overcoming the hardships that might come with them is doable. But most of all, that living MY life is what I need to do because the rewards are so great, and that trusting my instincts is really tapping into the person I was meant to be.

Barbara McCloskey

LIFE LESSONS # 5:
HONOR YOUR COMMITMENT TO YOURSELF

Recognizing your new priorities, reorienting your life and setting clear limits are essential building blocks for creating a life you love. However, keeping your word is also critical to this process. You must honor what you commit to and keep your promises, especially with yourself.

Unfortunately, women betray themselves more often than they do anyone else. You say one thing and do another. Any of you who have children (or for that matter who were once children) know how it feels to have a promise made and then not kept. You lose faith and trust in the other person. The same thing occurs with yourself. When you don't keep your word, you lose credibility with yourself, and it undermines your self-esteem. Every broken commitment is a crack in the foundation of a high quality life.

He has achieved success, who has lived well, laughed often, and loved much.

Bessie A. Stanley

How many times have you said you're going to exercise or eat better and not followed through? Have you noticed that the next time you try to make a similar promise to yourself it's tainted with doubt? You don't completely trust that you're going to do what you say.

Whatever you neglect to respect—the commitment to spend more time with your kids, to live by a financial budget, to be more understanding of your parents—these betrayals poison the well of your credibility. They undermine your integrity and trustworthiness. It's not that the fickle finger of fate is going to come down and punish you. It's about not having the internal support to accomplish the changes you want to make.

As life goes on it becomes tiring to keep up the character you invented for yourself, and so you relapse into individuality and become more like yourself every day. This is sometimes disconcerting for those around you, but a great relief to the person concerned.

Agatha Christie

Start small. Don't make any grand proclamations that will set you up for failure. Keep it simple. Only commit to what you honestly know you *can* and *will* do. Otherwise don't say it. For example, rather than proclaiming, "I'm going to exercise every day this week," say "I'm going to exercise for fifteen minutes today." It's the old Alcoholics Anonymous concept of one day at a time.

Instead of saying, "I'll never yell at my kids again," (which is next to impossible), why not say, "Today I'll speak to my children in a calm manner."

Or instead of saying, "From now on I'm going to spend at least a half an hour every day doing something that nurtures me," take the realistic approach of, "Today I'm going to set aside a half an hour for myself." The secret is to make promises that you know you can keep. Manageable commitments allow you to be successful and to become a person who keeps her word.

I am building trust and self-respect by keeping my commitments to myself.

Basic Tool: Daily Victory Log

At the end of every day, make a list of everything you've accomplished, acts of kindness, choices and achievements you are proud of both large and small. For example:

I exercised for an hour.

I didn't yell at my daughter, even though she didn't do her homework.

I brought my neighbor a pot of soup when she came home from the hospital.

Read your Victory Log at least once a week as a reminder of all your accomplishments, especially when you're feeling down or facing a difficult decision. By doing this you will recognize that your life has been a success and that the strengths you already have can support you in creating the life you want.

♨ The Finishing Touch

WHAT'S WORKING?

No matter how frazzled and worthless you may feel sometimes, there are certain things that *are* working in your life. So instead of dwelling on the negative, take a moment to consider what's working. Not only will you get a boost in self-confidence, you'll also see that you have a strong foundation upon which to build. There's no reason to fix what isn't broken.

It's time to grab a stack of paper, or even better your journal, and create a State of My Life Inventory.

Using a separate page for each, write down the following categories: relationships, family, money, health/well-being, career/job, social life, spiritual life/religion, leisure time and hobbies. Next make a list of everything you feel is going well in each of these areas. In some areas, you may not feel that anything is going right. Think again. No matter how small, there are always positives.

Now that you know what's working, turn to a new page and consider what's not working as well as you'd like. Be sure to go back over the same major areas. For example, if you are focusing on your family, you may realize that you're not spending as much time with your children as you'd like, or that you and your spouse haven't been out alone in over a month. Be honest with yourself. Pay attention to the quality of your life and not just the simple acts needed to survive each day. Now take charge of your life and make that dream a reality. It's fine to start small . . . but you have to start somewhere.

TAKE CARE OF YOURSELF

There is a connection
between self-nurturing and self-respect.

Julia Cameron

☕ Parking in the Center of the Garage

I've never lived alone until now. My mother, who made the decisions for the whole family, thought it was not proper for a young single woman to live alone, so I lived with her until I was married. My husband and I were married for fifty-one years, and although he was away many times during his army career, I had our children with me and was not living alone in the strictest sense.

When my husband died, our grandson lived in our home and remained with me for more than a year, but recently he decided he would make the responsible move out on his own. Now, at seventy- plus, I am living alone, in complete charge of my home, my cat, my car and myself. I can park on the left side of the garage, on the right, or in the position I prefer, smack in the middle.

I have learned that lunch can occur anywhere from 11 A.M. to 2:30 P.M., and can consist of a salad, a sandwich or popcorn. Dinner can be anytime from 4:30 to 10 P.M., and can feature such delicacies as meat and veggies, bacon and eggs, or even cheese and crackers. For those of us living alone, dinner is usually stir-fry, or the more properly labeled "one-dish meal." The important thing about dinnertime is that it should not interfere with my regular evening tryst with Tom Brokaw.

Living alone, I can eat fully dressed or in my pajamas and socks. My dining table is round with four chairs. I rotate my seating—sometimes on the north side, sometimes south, west or east. No sense sitting in the same chair all the time. This way I can see the dining room from all perspectives. No one is offended if I read or work a crossword puzzle while eating.

I haven't moved to the center of the bed, since my cat, Lucy, prefers the right side. Also, the radio is on the left, and judging from the few times Lucy has taken over the controls, her selection of music does not fit my taste, so I will maintain my claim to the left side.

Bedtime is another adjustment that has occurred in the household. I can snuggle in at nine or midnight. Who cares? If I awaken in the night, I can read or view a movie without disturbing anyone. Although I have learned that late, late shows on HBO or Showtime are a bit too risqué for my tastes, the American Movie Classics channel occasionally has a tearjerker from the '40s that suits me perfectly.

I have to admit there are some negative aspects to living alone, such as having to wait for company to come to move large pieces of furniture, eating the same meal two or three times until the leftovers are gone, having no one to hold the cat while I perform a delicate procedure with the clippers, and having to remove the dead bird from the dryer vent myself. There is also the gable that needs to be painted from the tall ladder, the lost key to the shed that I couldn't possibly have been responsible for, and the clock on the VCR that continues to show the wrong time. There is also the matter of how to retrieve the cotton in my ear from the failed cotton swab and the notes I've had to post on the basement walls identifying each fuse and the water turnoff. There is no one to remind me what it was I was going to write on my "to do" list, and no longer an excuse to buy cookies and ice cream.

However, the deodorant and hairspray are always where I left them. I have time for myself to contemplate things, even if I have forgotten what it was I planned to contemplate. I have, in fact, established a new identity—not daughter, wife, mother or grandmother, but a separate person in my own right—ME—still a work in progress.

Don't get me wrong; I love company and am thrilled when family or friends come for a short visit. But I really do love parking in the center of the garage.

Louise Hamm

Life Lesson #1:
Practice Self-Nurturing

Most women have been taught since childhood to put other people's needs first. In fact, much of your value as a woman has come from your ability to know what someone else needs. It's one of your talents. In fact, in our society one of the main qualities of being feminine is being selfless. Women have not only become comfortable with attending to others' needs, they've perfected the art.

When we truly care for ourselves, it becomes possible to care far more profoundly about other people. The more alert and sensitive we are to our own needs, the more loving and generous we can be towards others.

Eda LeShan

When women begin to bring themselves back into the picture, it frequently feels as if they're breaking an essential rule of femininity, like they're doing something forbidden. But think about it for a minute, if you don't take time to nurture yourself and recharge your battery, how can you truly care for others? You can't.

You wouldn't dream of driving your car when the gas gauge reads empty. You wouldn't think of asking your child to pull an all-nighter to prepare for final exams, yet you are continually pushing yourself past the breaking point and ignoring the fact that there will inevitably be negative repercussions to the continual denial of your needs.

Think back to the last time you were on an airplane. Remember the instructions the flight attendant gave when you were about to take off: "In case of an emergency, first place the oxygen mask securely around your nose and mouth and then place it on your child." The truth is, you have to come first—at least some of the time. This may make you uncomfortable, but think of it this way: Only to the extent that you love and take care of yourself are you able to love and take care of others.

Taking care of yourself is an essential part of creating a life you love. When you bring yourself back into the equation, you create a healthy balance in your life.

I come first, at least some of the time.

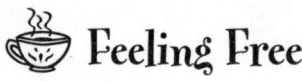 **Feeling Free**

> *There must be quite a few things a hot bath won't*
> *cure, but I don't know many of them.*

SYLVIA PLATH

I woke up feeling cranky. I didn't want to do housework, though the laundry was piling up. I didn't want to read the work I brought home from the office. I didn't want to do anything that resembled responsible behavior. It was that kind of day.

As I drank my morning tea, I thought I felt a headache coming on. Yes, there it was, a dull throb just behind my eyes. Maybe I should go back to bed until it subsided. As I put the dishes in the sink, it seemed that my muscles were beginning to ache. Or was the ache in my joints? That could mean I was coming down with the flu. Everyone I knew had the flu this year. Why should I be the one to escape it? I absolutely should be in bed.

I shuffled back to bed, wiggled under the covers and shut my eyes. Another couple of hours of sleep would be so nice, only I was now completely awake. I ought to get up.

But no, there was that headache and the beginning of a sniffle. Better get the tissues.

On my way back from the bathroom with a family-sized tissue box, I stopped to grab that big new novel I had bought but had no time to read. I opened the book and settled against the pillows.

The morning was moving along and so was my reading. Another twenty pages and I was stretching. I should try to crack the report I was working on. I should at least get up and do the wash. What if I was contagious? I certainly didn't want to spread any germs. The wash could wait. My family was resourceful enough to scrounge clothing for the next day.

Maybe I wasn't actually getting the flu. I didn't really want to be sick. To be truthful, all I wanted was a little time off. I needed to nurture myself away from people, chores, career and the outside world. Did I have to wait to be sick to do that? As a child, the only respite from school or family chores was illness. But I wasn't a child any more. Did I have to manufacture symptoms to provide myself with an excuse? No, I decided, I didn't.

I talked to myself. *Okay,* I said, *you need a day off. Admit it. Accept it. Toss out the guilt and enjoy a mini-vacation. What would you like to do? Read? You're already doing that. Pamper yourself? Take a bubble bath. Be a hermit? Let the machine answer the phone.*

I poured half the bottle of bath gel into the streaming

water and added a hearty handful of chamomile bath salts. Then I lit a vanilla-scented candle and gingerly stepped into the bathtub. With a grateful sigh, I immersed myself in my homemade spa. I heard the phone ring somewhere off in the distance and smiled.

Funny how the aches subsided in the heat of the tub. They just slipped away with the last of the bubbles down the drain. My head felt just fine, the throb replaced by a sense of well-being.

By late afternoon, I was back at it, refreshed physically, mentally and emotionally. And rather than feeling helpless, I felt empowered. I had given myself permission to listen and respond to my needs, to care for myself the way I tended to my family. I didn't need the crutch of illness to justify a rest. It was such a simple awareness, but then isn't it the simple things that set us free?

Ferida Wolff

LIFE LESSON #2: BANISH YOUR GUILT

Most women are caught in a tug-of-war between who they *think* they should be and who they are; between what they *want* to do and what they are actually able to do. In other words, you are at the mercy of your guilt demons. Your feelings of guilt often prevent you from taking care of yourself. Most of the time, these feelings stem from unrealistic expectations. You have impossible ideals that you strive to live up to—ideals such as, "I must always put other people's needs first," or "I should never disappoint anyone." These kinds of standards are not only impossible to meet, but they are harmful to your well-being.

Guilt is a major roadblock to taking care of yourself. There's always a list of things that have to be done that take precedence over attending to your own needs. Then there's the fear of who you'll disappoint if you occasionally make yourself a priority. But stop and consider for a moment that when you put yourself last on the list and allow guilt to run your life, the person who you continually disappoint is yourself.

Sometimes the most urgent and vital thing you can possibly do is take a complete rest.

Ashleigh Brilliant

Don't worry, there is something you can do—in fact, that you must do. Most of you have an idealized image of what good parents, good employees, good daughters, good wives should be, and are haunted by these images of perfection. Rather than confront the comparison between the idealized images and your actual self, many of you feel inadequate and guilt-ridden because you can't match up to your own impossibly high standards.

You have a choice, you can either adjust your standards so that they more closely match reality or you can change your behavior. In the majority of cases, we would suggest you get rid of those ludicrous expectations. Remember Super Woman? She's not dead—she never existed. It's time to admit that you are a mere human who has needs of her own.

For those of you who are parents, we have news for you. In case you haven't noticed, the times have changed. In the past, the "average" family meant a breadwinning father and a mother who stayed home with the children. Today, only 6 percent of families fit this description. In the majority of homes in America, both parents now work outside the home, even when there are children of preschool and elementary school age. Blended families and single-parent families are fast becoming the rule rather than the exception. Our roles have changed along with the demands made on us, yet our internal standards for ourselves often are not a practical match for our actual living situations.

If you are a mother and breadwinner, we challenge you to become realistic about what you can do in a day. You don't have to live up to the expectations of your mother, and you don't have to meet every demand of your children or husband.

I now create more realistic expectations and
I release all guilt about the things
I choose not to do.

☕ Life After Death

During the two months before my fortieth birthday I decided to really have a "feel sorry for myself" crying session. Then I made an appointment to see a doctor for my annual checkup. I asked to see a woman doctor. Surely a woman could do something for me. I was tired all the time, weighed about 200 pounds and was becoming more and more depressed.

The day came for my checkup. Mary Dailey, nurse practitioner, checked me for everything. She was wonderful. She told me that I had a good reason to be tired and she wanted to consider hospitalizing me. My blood count was low, my estrogen level was really bad. I was sixty pounds overweight, and on and on and on. Then and there I started taking iron, estrogen, calcium and daily vitamins. I call these my turning-forty meds. I told her I would start an exercise program right away. "Oh, no you don't," she said. "Not until we get all of this other stuff in order. You're not going to be able to handle an exercise class for awhile." I made an appointment to see her in another three months.

Three months went by and I couldn't wait for Mary

Dailey to release me. I visited our local kickboxing and Tae Bo exercise center and bought all the equipment. I paid the $200 yearly fee for a brand-new start on a brand-new me. Or so I thought. Ms. Dailey still didn't think it was such a good idea for me to start just yet. "Not yet. Things are looking better but your iron deficiency is still there." Her words burst my bubble. *Come on, I'm over forty and things are looking pretty thick and saggy,* I thought to myself. It was horrible but I had to wait.

The next doctor's appointment was three months later. I was released to start an exercise program. *Great,* I thought. *This is going to be awesome. In six months I should weigh about 140 pounds and look ten years younger.* I put on my sweats, wrapped my hands, grabbed my towel and boxing gloves and headed to my kickboxing class.

These classes are incredible. The first row is 100- to 120-pounders. The second row is your 125- to 150-pounders and in the very back are your overheated, out of breath, out of shape, not keeping up, 160- to 200-pounders. Halfway through the class, I was dying. I dragged myself to the car coughing and fighting for breath. I could barely drive. I got home and lay on the floor. I couldn't move for two hours. *Okay, okay,* I told myself. *I'll be like this for a couple of weeks.* I tried to convince myself things would get better.

By week three, I had worked myself up to a half-hour before I left the building wheezing, crawling to my car. I decided this wasn't going to work. I was six pounds lighter, but I couldn't stand the idea of facing another class. That was it! Six months of waiting to start this stupid class and now I just couldn't go on. What was going to happen to me? I didn't want to give up. But the thought of exercising to TV and tapes just didn't motivate me.

Then I had an idea. When I was in college, I was an aerobics instructor. What if I got together with a couple of friends to work out? I knew the perfect place for our workout: the Salvation Army Recreation Center. I visited Judy Ponce, the social services coordinator. She gave me permission to use their facility. The last week of August 2000, I started exercising with seven other ladies every Monday, Wednesday and Friday. I worked hard putting low-impact, high-energy routines together. However, this wasn't the most difficult part of the class. I felt intimidated. I wondered, *How can I lead an aerobics class looking like this?* I realized my attitude needed healing as much as my health. I wasn't the best qualified, but I was willing. Before long, the Salvation Army was getting calls asking about the class and we started to see our numbers grow.

For the new year, I decided to place a small classified ad "FREE Aerobics Class" to encourage people to keep their fitness resolutions. I drove up to the center on January 3, 2001. I thought the Salvation Army had planned an event on my exercise night and forgot to tell me. I couldn't even find a parking place. There were so many people. As I unlocked the door, I turned around and asked, "Is everybody here for the exercise class?" I got seventy yeses. Can you believe it? Seventy people started exercising with me.

So here I am, celebrating one year. I am forty pounds lighter. My energy and self-esteem have climbed through the roof. The local news did a story on it and people talk about it to me wherever I go. My husband said he called for his prescription and they asked him if Rita Williams was his wife. They told him that I was their aerobics instructor. I have been asked to do demonstrations for the hospital health fair. The local diet programs refer their clients to me.

Not long ago, I had an interview for a job. The woman interviewing me said, "So, you're Rita. I've heard so much about you and your exercise classes. You'll never realize how many women's lives you have impacted."

There are now more than 250 women enrolled. I now instruct eight classes a week. We have two more volunteer instructors and a volunteer that provides childcare. These women held a fund-raiser. They bought the class a brand-new stereo and a ton of new music.

With our one-year celebration, we chose a name for our class: CardioJam with Rita. . . . Hold that tummy tight, tight, tight!

Rita V. Williams

LIFE LESSON #3:
GET PHYSICAL

How many times have you heard, "You just need to eat right and exercise"? It's become the mantra for our health-conscious culture. But for most of us it sounds like we're being sentenced to a life of hard labor: pumping iron and sweating away on the StairMaster plus boring eating—broccoli, low-fat cottage cheese, broiled chicken. Doesn't sound like much fun. Investing in your health has to become more of a journey toward well-being and less of a task if you're going to make this a lifelong commitment.

Many women take their bodies for granted. They burn the proverbial candle at both ends. They eat fast food, only move when absolutely necessary and expect that there won't be any consequences to their neglect. But there are. Maybe not immediately, especially if you're in your twenties or thirties when you still have a warranty on your body, but sooner or later it's going to expire and your disregard for your health is going to catch up with you. Think about it for a minute: Would you drive your car with the oil light flashing? Not likely. Would you put low-grade fuel in a Ferrari? Never. However, amazingly, we all too often abuse

Incredibly, many of
you think nothing
of spending hours
researching and then
days or weeks shop-
ping for a new car or
an appliance for your
home. But you find it
difficult to carve out
30 minutes a day to do
something that will
improve your health.
Don't wait until you
get a wake-up call in
the form of an illness
to begin taking care
of your body. Make
exercise an unshakable
priority.

and ignore our most precious vehicle.

Your physical health is fundamental. Your body is the vehicle through which you express yourself and your life. When something's wrong with your body, when you're in pain or feeling out of sorts, you can bet that everything else in your life is affected. Your health needs to be one of your top priorities. Caring for your body is critical to living a high quality life. When you're in a state of optimal health, just about everything else in your life is better. But like everything else, this requires effort. For those of you who have ignored your bodies, now's the time to rediscover them.

*My physical well-being is essential
to my sense of fulfillment
and I am making
my health a priority.*

☕ If I Were Lucky

If I were lucky in this lifetime, I would learn the art of letting go.

I would start with the bathroom scale, that little square joy buster. Gone!

Next would be my watch, keeper of rigid rituals and joyless appointments. Gone!

Perfection, next big hit. Let the housework pile up and invite lots of friends over. Just put the vacuum cleaner in the middle of the living room and leave it there for six months.

Next, get rid of that worry dance I do. The health of my husband, the safety of my children, not enough money, what people think, being alone, not being alone, terrorists, tax collectors, termites . . . get a grip! Let it go.

I would travel the world and take lots of black and white photos of all the wonderful faces.

I would sit on the beach with my friends and eat junky hot dogs.

I would take long walks with my husband through the village to the lighthouse.

Sometimes I would sit quietly on my porch and listen to the birds for hours. Sometimes I would put on jazz or opera and turn it up really loud.

I would surround myself with people who love nature, laughter and dessert.

I would spend my time living large and doing nothing.

I would sit back and enjoy the journey.

Avis Drucker

LIFE LESSON #4:
CULTIVATE A NURTURING VOICE

One essential aspect of self-nurturing is to cultivate a compassionate attitude toward yourself. Women tend to be critical and hard on themselves, when this is the last thing they need. What you really need is a more positive, loving attitude toward yourself. Unfortunately, most women are experts at supporting and being understanding of other people, but when it comes to themselves they fail miserably.

Perfectionism is the voice of the oppressor, the enemy of the people. It will keep you cramped and insane your whole life.

Anne Lamott

Everyone has an inner critic sitting on their shoulder watching and judging their every move. Do any of these phrases sound familiar? "You look old, even your earlobes have wrinkles." "If your head weren't attached, you'd probably forget that, too." "Try as you might, you are never going to amount to anything." The sad truth is, most women continually have this kind of running dialogue with themselves.

Have you ever noticed that no matter what you do, your critic is never satisfied? Nothing you do seems to please her or, more importantly, gets her to shut up. Would you want a friend who was constantly critical of you, blamed you for everything that went wrong, put you down no matter what you did, kept a running tally of all your failures, and beat you up for even the smallest mistakes? Not if she were the last person alive. And yet you repeatedly give in to this tyrant.

Those who are lifting the world upward and onward are those who encourage more than criticize.

Elizabeth Harrison

When you feel discouraged, depressed and self-hating, your critic has you in her grips. It's impossible to feel good about yourself when there is a voice in your head continually telling you what you're doing is wrong or how bad you are. It's time to take charge, to bring in your positive, protective, nurturing voice.

But how do you start to cultivate a compassionate voice? First send your inner critic on an all-expenses-paid vacation to the Bahamas. Get her off your case.

Now develop that nurturing inner voice. This is a voice that will reassure you when you feel overwhelmed. "It's okay

Questions Worth Asking

- What am I most critical of about myself?
- What is the most positive thing I can think of in response to that criticism?
- What might happen if I started to concentrate on my positive qualities and strengths?

that the bill can't be paid today, you have a paycheck coming on Friday." This is the voice that will give you a lift when you need it. "You may have gained a few pounds, but you still look great!" This is a voice that will encourage you to take time for yourself when you need it. "Yes, you deserve to read your book now." And this is a voice that will put your expectations and those of others in perspective. "You cook a lot of great meals, so tonight it's perfectly fine to just stop and pick something up."

The more you use your nurturing voice, the stronger it will become. Even if it feels a bit awkward at first, continue to incorporate your supportive voice into your everyday life.

Remember, it may take time before your nurturing voice begins to dominate your internal dialogue. However, over time your compassionate voice will overcome your inner critic. What a relief this will be! As you make more space for yourself on the inside, you'll also have an easier time creating space in your everyday life.

I deserve the praise and support of my compassionate inner voice.

Basic Tool: Strengthen Your Defender

Take an $8\frac{1}{2}$"x 11" sheet of paper and fold it down the center. Make two columns: one for your critical voice and one for your nurturing, compassionate voice. Then, without censoring, write the critical statements you frequently make about yourself. Let it all out.

Now, imagine someone who accepts you just the way you are, a parent, grandparent, friend. If you can't think of an actual person, imagine how it would feel to have someone like that standing next to you. Feel the warmth and acceptance from this person. Now in the other column write your positive, defending, compassionate responses to all those critical statements. Allow your nurturing voice to have her say.

Here's an example of how it works:

Critical Voice: You think you deserve some time for yourself? How about the laundry piled in the corner or the bills that are unpaid.

Nurturing Voice: None of those things are urgent. I deserve some time for myself.

Critical Voice: Yeah, me, me, me. You're just another selfish crybaby.

Nurturing Voice: No I'm not. I work hard and the majority of the time I'm responsible, but I need a break.

Critical Voice: You don't know what hard work is.

Nurturing Voice: Yes I do. I run errands all day, make sure the house is in order, the kids get to school and make sure that their homework is done. If you have something to say, you'll have to say it in a nicer way or I don't want to hear it.

Now tear that piece of paper in half and throw away the negative half. It's time to begin to banish your inner critic.

🍵 Sticks and Stones

"Sticks and stones may break my bones, but words can never hurt me."

Once upon a time, my friend Joan believed that childhood chant. At least, she tried to. When she was young. And plump. And constantly being teased.

Then things changed. Joan grew up—and out.

As an adult, she tips the scales at well over 500 pounds. Her friends politely say she's . . . "heavy." Her doctor calls her "morbidly obese." The rest of the world calls her *fat*.

Some people whisper the word. Some people say it out loud, to her face. And, believe it or not, there are some people who say things even worse.

Don't think she hasn't heard the words. She has. And they hurt. Deeply. But Joan has learned how to avoid the cutting remarks: She simply avoids the people who make them. She stays home.

In her house.

Where it's safe.

But with their twenty-fifth wedding anniversary approaching, her husband planned a romantic evening for

the two of them. An evening out. Knowing it would be difficult—to Joan's way of thinking, the only thing worse than
being in public was *eating* in public—Dan, nevertheless,
began a persuasive campaign to convince Joan that she
must join him for dinner at a nice restaurant. She agreed.

Reluctantly.

Warily.

To distract herself from fretting about the impending
event, Joan, an accomplished seamstress, decided to sew a
dressy new blouse for their celebration.

Then, all too soon, the big night arrived.

Dan had chosen wisely. The lighting was romantic, the
ambiance sweet, the wait-staff attentive. The food was out-
of-this-world delicious. The restaurant was perfect.
Unfortunately, the patrons weren't.

Joan managed to ignore the blunt comments. She even
managed to disregard the rude stares. But she couldn't
overlook the young girl at the table across from them. The
youngster never took her eyes off Joan. When the girl stood
up and headed toward their table, Joan cringed.
Experience had taught her that kids could be especially
cruel.

The wide-eyed little girl paused next to Joan. Reaching
out a single, tentative finger, she touched Joan's indigo
velvet blouse.

"You're soft and cuddly, like my bunny," she said.

Joan held her breath while a tiny hand gently stroked her sleeve.

"You're so pretty in that top." The little girl smiled and walked back to her seat.

A simple comment; a single compliment. That was all. But, according to Joan, it was enough to change her life and to alter her perspective.

"Now," Joan says, "when people stare—why, I immediately recall miniature angel fingers caressing me. And I'm certain everyone is merely . . . admiring my outfit."

"Now," Joan says, "when people mutter behind my back—why, I swear I can hear a young angel's voice reminding me that I'm pretty. And I'm equally sure the words everyone whispers are . . . flattering."

"That's all I hear—now," Joan says. "Only compliments. Words that can never hurt me."

Carol McAdoo Rehme

LIFE LESSON #5:
ACCEPT COMPLIMENTS

People talk about someone being conceited, getting a swelled head or being stuck on themselves. You've been discouraged from not only singing your own praises, but from accepting compliments. How many times has someone paid you a compliment and you simply accepted it? Probably rarely, if ever.

In most cases, you make excuses and give a litany of reasons why you don't deserve the compliment. Someone tells you you're a good cook and you immediately respond, "Oh, it was nothing." A friend comments on how nice you look and you say, "You must be kidding. Me? My hair is a disaster." When you reject someone's compliment, you're in effect discounting the other person as well as yourself.

How do you respond when a friend gives you a gift? Are you appreciative? Do you express your gratitude? A compliment is a verbal gift. Accept it graciously and allow it to sink in.

It's time to stop eating humble pie. We must become more comfortable with receiving these flattering remarks. Let yourself enjoy the friendly praise of others. The next time someone pays you a compliment, practice saying "Thank you." Nothing more. Don't worry, you're in no danger of becoming conceited.

I receive compliments with openness and grace.

The Dear Stand

"A deer stand. That's what I want for my birthday."

Diane stood beside the washing machine surrounded by piles of laundry that never seemed to grow smaller. A sink full of dirty dishes awaited her in the kitchen, and toys were scattered everywhere. The phone was ringing, the dog was barking, the twins were sword fighting with sticks in the middle of the family room.

Why her husband Paul thought this was a good time to bring up the subject of her birthday, she couldn't fathom, but she'd been planning this answer for a long time.

"A deer stand?" Paul looked at her as though she'd lost her mind.

"When did you take up hunting?"

"I haven't taken up hunting. I just want you to build me a deer stand in that tree." She pointed to the giant maple that graced the far corner of their suburban backyard. "And it needs to have a rope ladder—one that I can pull in after me once I'm up there."

Paul walked away shaking his head, and Diane heard him mumble something about being wrong all these years to think that women wanted gifts of perfume or jewelry or lingerie.

"A deer stand," he muttered over and over. "She wants a deer stand."

How could she possibly make him understand her need to have a quiet spot of her own? She craved a place where she could escape—if only for a few minutes—from the never-ending demands of running a household and raising three small boys, a place that was hers and hers alone, a place designed to make it impossible to do anything at all except relax.

Many of the men in her family—including Paul—were deer hunters, and she had always envied them their private time high above the forest floor where nothing was required except patience and quiet.

Last winter, during hunting season, an idea had dawned on her. She could have that special time and place, too, without becoming a hunter or even leaving home. All she needed was a deer stand of her own.

How could she explain that to Paul?

But he never asked for an explanation. He simply came home on the afternoon of her birthday with a load of lumber and a box of nails and hollered up the stairs to the boys.

"Come on down, fellas, and let's build your mom a birthday present!" Paul Jr., age eleven, and nine-year-olds Kyle and Seth clambered down the steps and into the yard where they busied themselves measuring and sawing and hammering until it was nearly dark.

Under no circumstance was Diane to come out or even take a peek into the backyard.

Paul finally came inside and took her by the hand. "Close your eyes," he said, "and come with me." The late afternoon breeze blew cool against her skin as he led her out the back door. She could hear the boys giggling.

"Now you can look," Paul said when they reached the far corner of the yard. "Happy Birthday!"

It was beautiful. Nestled in the crook of a sturdy tree branch about ten feet above the ground, the deer stand was just the right size for one person. A safety rail surrounded its deck, and from it hung a soft rope ladder.

Paul and the boys were grinning like they'd burst. "Aren't you gonna try it out, Mom?" Seth asked.

"Why sure I am." With that, Diane grabbed hold of the ladder and made her way up. She plopped into the lawn chair that had been set on the platform. "Perfect!" she declared. "Just exactly what I had in mind."

"And look at this, Mom," Kyle shouted from below. "A pulley with a bucket, so you can take your stuff up with you." Paul Jr. placed a package tied with a huge pink bow into the bucket and Diane hauled it up.

Inside the package was a wooden sign. On it, the words

MOM'S DEAR STAND had been painstakingly carved. Paul winked at her as she read the sign aloud, and tears welled up in her eyes.

"Thanks, guys. It's the best birthday present I've ever gotten."

And it turned out she was right. Whenever the piles of dirty clothes or dirty dishes seemed to overwhelm her, whenever she couldn't bear listening to the telephone or the television or three rowdy boys for one more minute, whenever she felt a desperate need to escape, she'd remember the birthday present waiting for her in the backyard.

Then she'd fill a bottle with tea, drop a handful of cookies into a sandwich bag, and grab a book or magazine that she'd been trying to find the time to read. She'd load those things into her bucket and make her way up the rope ladder to the platform in the crook of the maple tree.

Sometimes she stayed for an hour or two, snacking and reading or even catching a catnap. Sometimes she stayed only a few minutes, just long enough to still the pounding of her heart by saying a little prayer or watching a mother bird tend to the babies in her nest.

The boys knew that when Mom was in the deer stand with the rope ladder pulled up, they were not to bother her.

The phone could ring, the drier could buzz, the television could go haywire, and soggy Cheerios could harden and dry in the bottom of cereal bowls. None of those things mattered when Diane was having her quiet time in the tree.

She always descended renewed and refreshed, ready to take on with energy and patience anything her hectic, wonderful life could throw at her.

MOM'S DEAR STAND, the letters carved in her sign said. She'd never forget how Paul had winked the first time she'd read those words. "I didn't have the heart to tell them they'd spelled 'deer' wrong," he whispered to her later.

She shook her head. "They didn't spell it wrong at all," she whispered back. "It's the dearest present anyone has ever given me. They spelled it exactly right."

Jennie Ivey

LIFE LESSON # 6:
SCHEDULE TIME JUST FOR YOU

Many women feel that time for themselves is stolen time in which they are playing hooky from more important endeavors! It's time to stop feeling that you have to get sick in order to take time for yourself. It's time to start scheduling self-nurturing activities, because when you schedule personal time you make it legitimate.

Take a mini-vacation. We all need a break from our busy lives. We know, there's so much to do, you couldn't possibly take time just for yourself. But let's put things in perspective. There is very little in life that requires your immediate attention. You may think that it does, but with rare exceptions, most things can wait until tomorrow. In other words, take time for yourself.

Your health and well-being may be in jeopardy if you're neglecting yourself. And if you're running on empty, you're not doing anyone any good, least of all yourself. You may be going through the motions of living, but sleepwalking through life doesn't exactly qualify as creating a life you love.

Too many of us are hung up on what we don't have, can't have, or won't ever have. We spend too much energy being down, when we could use that same energy—if not less of it—doing, or at least trying to do, some of the things we really want to do.

Terry McMillan

Fantasize about what time for yourself would be like. What do you want to do? Where do you want to go? Who, if anyone, do you want to spend this time with?

Start small, do what feels manageable—a lunch date with a friend, cuddling up for an hour with a good book, an afternoon at the movies, a walk in the woods, spending part of a day under the covers, napping, watching your favorite movie, or having a picnic in the park. The possibilities are endless.

If you really want to be daring, take an entire day off. This doesn't mean catching up on unpaid bills, doing work at home or running errands. It's a day devoted to you and you alone. Let your family know that you're going to take some time just for you. Notify your office that you're going to take a mental health day. Take a sick day without being sick. Use one of your vacation days just to pamper yourself.

Be courageous and schedule at least one hour of personal time at least once a week. Remember, it can be something as simple as getting up before your family to enjoy your morning coffee or tea in peace, soaking in a bubble bath surrounded by candlelight, or watching the petals open on the roses in your garden.

Questions Worth Asking

- If you took time for yourself, what three things would you do?

- Now choose one of those activities and make a commitment to do it within the next month.

When scheduling personal time, keep it simple. The fewer details the better. One way to guard against the tyranny of the "shoulds" is to make a plan with a friend. By using the buddy system, you are less likely to cancel your date.

It takes as much energy to wish as it does to plan.

Eleanor Roosevelt

Self-care is essential. It's necessary for your psychological, emotional and physical well-being. When you set aside time just for you, you're declaring your self-worth. In return, other people will value you and treat you with greater respect.

Taking care of yourself isn't a reward for completing your "to do" list. It's a function of the fact that you're a human being and you deserve nurturing every single day. Caring for yourself is your birthright; have the courage to claim it. Our challenge in a society that worships accomplishment and abhors idleness is to learn when to "do" and when to "be." Discovering how to find a balance between the two is essential to your well-being.

I like myself enough
to spend time with myself.

☕ A Lasting Impression

I pulled into the driveway and parked my car after making a quick trip through the supermarket. As the car door swung open, I grabbed one grocery bag under each arm, stood up, and used my hips to close the door. Seeing that my arms were full, my teenage son Robert stopped his phone conversation long enough to open the kitchen door. Once inside, I hurriedly put away the frozen flounder, red snapper and halibut that were on special at the meat market. After putting the rest of the groceries away in the pantry, I folded the paper sacks and placed them in the recycling bin. Looking at my watch, I noted that my husband Fred would be home soon and started preparing dinner.

A few minutes later, Fred came home from work with a curious look on his face. "Have the boys been playing basketball today?" he inquired.

"No, why do you ask?" I answered.

"There's a large dent in the rear passenger door of the car about the size of a basketball," he said in anger.

My face turned red, and I swallowed hard, "Really?"

"Would I kid you about something like that? Come and

see for yourself." Fred turned on his heel and walked out the kitchen door.

I turned off the stove, wiped my hands on a paper towel and followed him outside to assess the damage. Sure enough, the rear passenger door had a huge dent in it.

"Are you sure the boys haven't been shooting hoops today? See this dent? It looks like a basketball hit the car door!" he said.

Tears welled up in my eyes. My face flushed. I sheepishly admitted that my "basketball buttocks" had dented the door.

Fred's eyes widened, "How'd you do that?"

"Well, with my hands full of groceries, I sort of used my backside to bump the car door shut," I confessed.

Fred shook his head and examined the car more closely. He winked at me as he measured my hips with his hands. With his hands held apart, he turned toward the car door. It was a perfect match. My heart sank. The visual was a depressing reality.

Fred found the toilet plunger in the garage and began working on the dented door. About that time, Robert reappeared.

"Mom, when's dinner?" Then he noticed his dad. "Whatcha doin'?"

"You'd never believe it if I told you, son."

The suction of the plunger popped the dent from the door. Fortunately, there was no permanent damage, except to my ego.

Relieved, I said, "Oh, thank God! I'm so embarrassed!"

Suddenly, I started to giggle. The laughter was contagious and uncontrollable. We both held our sides as we howled. My son, convinced we were both totally out of our minds, went back into the house shaking his head in disbelief.

"Well, I never would have expected *this* when I came home," Fred said with a belly laugh.

"I'm sorry. I won't do it again," I replied with a chuckle.

Afterwards, I thought how kind Fred had been not to tease me in front of the children. Instead, Fred chose to treat this incident as a private joke. I remembered the times I criticized my children in front of others or laughed at their childhood antics, perhaps unintentionally bruising their self-esteem. I vowed I'd pay attention, be more aware of my actions and reactions, always hold my family in high regard and think the best of them—even in the worst of circumstances.

The car door survived, my ego recovered after weeks of dieting, but my husband's loving kindness made a lasting impression on me!

Sharla Taylor

LIFE LESSON #7:
CULTIVATE A SENSE OF HUMOR

Laughter is healing. A good laugh is therapeutic. Did you know that when you laugh your brain secretes chemicals that act as antidepressants? Laughter even gives your immune system a boost. It's a great stress reducer. When you laugh, your brain releases endorphins that create feelings of joy and euphoria. There's nothing like a good laugh to break the intensity of a situation and give you some much needed perspective.

Having a sense of humor is another facet of investing in your health. Yet, in the midst of our hectic routines we too often forget to laugh. We become so serious that we lose touch with our sense of joy and become somber and stale, neither of which is good for our overall sense of well-being.

We've all had days when nothing seems to go right. We want things to be a certain way and we just can't make it happen. One of the greatest benefits of having a sense of humor is if you can laugh, you can get through anything. You simply can't laugh and be stressed at the same time. You have a choice. You can allow yourself to become more and more uptight or you can accept things as they are and lighten up. Ask yourself if you take yourself and your life too seriously.

You've probably had the experience of being able to laugh at yourself even in the midst of a difficult or frustrating situation and the relief that brings. Make a point of lightening up. Start to see the humor in the ironies of everyday life. The next time you're faced with a dilemma, add a pinch of humor. Inevitably you'll feel better. Remember, when all else fails, laugh.

I laugh easily and often.

⚔ The Finishing Touch

••

WHAT DO YOU REALLY WANT FOR YOURSELF?

This is a self-care inventory. It's just for you—no one else needs to see it, so there's no one to impress. It's simply a way for you to assess how well you're taking care of yourself.

Take a moment and answer the following questions:

1. How often do you take time to do something fun each week?
   ○ At least once a week   ○ Rarely   ○ Never

2. When was the last time you took time to be with a friend, had a massage, or did something purely nurturing for yourself?
   ○ Last week   ○ Last month   ○ I can't remember

3. How often do you do some form of physical exercise?
   ○ At least twice a week   ○ Sporadically
   ○ Almost never

4. What do you do to unwind and relax?
   ○ Watch TV   ○ Go for a walk   ○ Have a glass of wine

5. How do you feel about your body? Do you like the way you look? On a scale of 1–5 (1, being you hate your body; 5, you love it.)

○ 1 ○ 2 ○ 3 ○ 4 ○ 5

6. Are you within ten pounds of your ideal weight?
○ Yes ○ No

7. How often do you feel irritable because you are over-stressed and exhausted?
○ At least once a week ○ Every day
○ Only occasionally

8. Do you ask for help when you need it?
○ Often ○ Rarely ○ Never

9. Do you have as much physical contact and nurturing as you would like?
○ Yes ○ No

10. How often do you say yes when you want to say no?
○ Often ○ Rarely ○ Never

11. Are you doing what you want to be doing with your life?
○ Yes ○ No

12. Do you look forward to coming home at the end of the day?
○ Yes ○ No

13. When was the last time you laughed?
    ◯ Recently   ◯ I can't remember

14. How much time do you have each week just to relax?
    ◯ Plenty   ◯ Very little   ◯ None

Once you've had a chance to answer the above questions, think about how well you're doing in terms of taking care of yourself. On a scale of 1–10 (1, absolutely abominable and neglectful; 10, terrific), rate how you are doing with your own self-care.

Utterly neglected 1 2 3 4 5 6 7 8 9 10 Well cared for

Please be honest with yourself. Remember, this is just between you and you.

Essential Ingredient #4

SURROUND YOURSELF
WITH SUPPORT

Call it a clan, call it a network,
call it a tribe, call it a family.
Whatever you call it, whoever you are,
you need one.

Jane Howard

Granny's Ninth Birthday

*I often think, how could I have survived
without these women?*

CLAUDETTE RENNER

I stood at my front door surrounded by balloons as each friend handed me a colorful package. "Happy Birthday, Twink!" With a childlike curtsey I thanked them.

"Are any b-o-y-s coming?" asked Becky, my redheaded friend.

"No way!" shouted Ruth, "This is just for girls." Ruth is 5'10" and very opinionated.

These were friends I'd known a long time. Becky's hair is red; she dyes the gray. Ruth has been 5'10" for sixty of her seventy-two years.

Eight members of our Granny Group had come to celebrate a little-girl birthday, one of many parties I missed growing up. My mother died nineteen days before my sixth birthday. Devastated, my father moved us to another state so we could live with his parents. I overheard my father and grandmother decide to simply skip my birthday, thinking I would not be aware of that day. My six-year-old mind concluded they didn't think I was worth celebrating. That was the first of the birthday parties I didn't have.

On this, my fifty-ninth birthday, secure in my adulthood, I asked this treasured group of friends to help me celebrate my ninth birthday.

Some guests quickly snapped the paper hats on their heads and blew their party blowers at the prissy ones who adjusted the elastic over their hairdos.

Children play games at parties, and we weren't to be outdone. Cat, who had just had a hip replacement, managed to get down on her knees to join in a game of jacks around our rugged old six-foot coffee table. Genea went first. She got all the way to the threesies only because she had played with her grandkids the week before. When Myrna bounced the ball, it flew across the table. We let her try again and again until she finally picked up all the jacks in onesies. Then it was Patti's turn. When she missed, she glared at Myrna. "Look what you made me do," she sassed.

"You started it!" replied Myrna, flowing into a nine-year-old attitude. Becky, who spends much of her time speaking to women's groups, crumpled to the floor laughing.

"Enough's enough," I giggled. "Let's eat the ice cream and cake."

The pretend nine-year-olds grunted and moaned as we

helped each other back to a standing position. Gladly we went to the dining room table, a place where our bodies felt much more at home.

Duncan Hines had helped me make a great chocolate cake as I pretended to be both my mother and my nine-year-old self. I knew it was good—because I ate a chunk that stuck in the pan. The white frosting had stood in lovely peaks—until I tried to decorate it. It was supposed to say "Happy Birthday, Twink" in yellow, red and blue. My handiwork caused purples, greens and oranges to swirl with the primary colors in a mass of modern art. When Becky brought in the cake, I announced, "I made it myself!"

Everyone sang "Happy Birthday" to me. The joy of all my should-have-been birthdays welled up in a childlike excitement. They sang to me because they loved me. On my birthday we celebrated me.

I had never felt worthy enough for anyone to bring me a gift. Now, with all this attention, I knew my true friends had spent time and money on me. Cautiously I reached for a present. "Open the big one first," Patti demanded.

Did she know it was from my husband? Slowly, with a growing sense of wonder, I took off the ribbon and wrapping paper with pictures of baby dolls. My eyes opened wide. A Betsy Wetsy! I fumbled to get her out of the box and then held her tight. My own doll! She wasn't soft, but oh, she cuddled so well. It was difficult to let her go. My adult took over and I knew it was right to pass her around.

"Don't give her milk because it makes her stink." Ruth wrinkled up her nose and made us all nine again.

"Open mine next."

"No, mine's right here."

Each present had a kid's card and a personal note. The card on the sticker kit said, "Because I love you! Stick to who you are."

Becky's card read, "To a child who has grown up to be God's precious princess." After I unwrapped the big box, I found a gift wrapped in grown-up paper. It contained a plastic silver tiara with a huge pretend sapphire in the center. For the rest of the afternoon I was a princess.

As the party came to a close, each girl drew a favor out of the "favor box" in the center of the table. The little figurines were suitable for girls—or for women who want to remember being girls for a day.

"Twink, you're a great nine-year-old. This was such fun." The grannies shared hugs all around.

Becky hugged the princess. "Thanks for letting us play a part in your healing. You are radiant."

That day a forgotten part of me grew up. The message children learn from their birthday parties is now mine. I am valuable and worth celebrating.

Twink DeWitt

Life Lesson #1:
Build Lasting Friendships

As the previous story so wonderfully illustrates, we all need to have people in our lives with whom we share the good times and who support us through the challenges we will inevitably face. We need people in our lives who share our dreams, help us conquer our fears, make us laugh and provide a safe space in which we can explore and grow. We need friends who hold the thread of our shared history, and who in times of doubt remind us of our best, most authentic self.

When you approach the end of your life what will be among your most cherished memories? Will it be how successful you were on the job? How much money you had in the bank? The size of the house you lived in or the kind of car you drove? Most likely not. What you want is to remember and be remembered for how much love you shared in your life. You want to leave this Earth knowing that you touched other people and

A friend doesn't go on a diet because you are fat. A friend never defends a husband who gets his wife an electric skillet for her birthday. A friend will tell you she saw your old boyfriend and he's a priest.

Erma Bombeck

- Who makes me feel valuable and worth celebrating?
- What kind of support do I get from them?
- Who do I talk to when I'm upset?
- When was the last time I made time to connect with the people I find valuable and worth celebrating?
- What can I do to provide support to them?
- When will I take these actions?

allowed yourself to have deep, meaningful relationships. You want to know that you made a contribution and left the world a better place. These are the things that truly matter.

Unfortunately, it's easy to neglect this vital area of your life. You can so easily allow your friendships to fall to the bottom of your "to do" list. You overlook the very people on whom you most depend. As a result, your life becomes more stressful and lacks the depth and richness that only significant relationships can provide.

Creating a network of support takes time, but it's time well spent. While there are some friendships that can sustain a lack of contact, most important relationships require an investment of time and attention. Nurture your friendships, so when you need them, they're there.

I am making my friendships a priority and devoting myself to nurturing these connections.

☕ "Best" Truths

The most precious moments in friendship
were not when I laughed with a friend, though
those times are so good!, but when I cried
with a friend and she reached out
and listened and understood.

FRAN MORGAN

Years ago, "the group" meant everything to me. They defined my thoughts and my behaviors for fifteen years, and then, I lost my husband. He died slowly, at forty-two, of a bad heart. After the excruciating horror was over, the great slog through the days began. Along with tending two small daughters, a strange me began to emerge—a person who, like the clouds—was changing.

"Pick yourself up, girl, or lie down and die!" I huffed, to which was also added, "Tell 'em the blunt truth!" I used my then version of truth, which unfortunately took the form of ax bludgeoning, accompanied by other strange acts—including a very strange me.

"The group" dropped me. I didn't understand why,

because I needed them desperately. Truth was, I was a real nut case, who didn't even recognize herself. It broke my heart, because I thought these friends were forever. Worse still, we never talked about it, confronted each other, aired it, let it all hang out. Something. Anything. They were just gone. It left an inner black hole that exists for me even to this day because it's unfinished.

At that time, down the block lived Linda who was not big in my life and certainly not a part of "the group." She was someone who seemed to simply like the heck out of me, but the other group took up such a huge space in my heart, the friendship hadn't gone past the sprouting stage.

One day, she came over. I don't know what happened, but all of a sudden we were fighting about how to raise our four girls. It escalated, heated, turned to a shouting match, then exploded, because she injected something about me dropping "THE" group. Me! I picked up a chair; she put up her fists. I hollered for her to "get out of my house!"

I told her if she wouldn't go, I'd leave my own house, and I did. I ended up sitting on the ground of my backyard. She followed me out there to try and talk. I bawled, completely undone. Eventually, she left.

The other group had dropped me, now Linda had too. Confused, I sank into a series of warped and solitary Isabel "truths," sprinkled with salt to be rubbed on demand into self-righteous wounds.

One morning, weeks later, after our kids had gone to school—they always walked together and hadn't the slightest idea that we'd had such a fight—the doorbell rang. It was Linda. As soon as I answered, she ran down to the end of the sidewalk. "I don't know what's the matter with you! I don't understand you!" she hollered, hands on her hips. "I can't understand all this changing you're doing. I don't know what's the matter with me either, but I know that I love you, want you in my life, and I'm not giving up!"

I just stood looking through the screen, dumbstruck by her words: "I love you."

She started marching back toward her house. I opened the door, and cautiously sidestepped down into my front yard.

"Wait!" I called.

We came together. Slowly.

"You dropped those friends," she stated, with a shaking voice. "I'm scared I'll be next."

"I didn't drop them!" I rasped. "They dropped me!"

Now sitting close in the front yard, what followed was the airing of our best truths, from the heart, shared softly. That day, we planted our feet firmly on the friendship path, never to be parted again.

Over the years, I've had friends who've stuck through the best and worst of times, like Linda. I've had friends who've just gone away. I've had words with close friends and grown away from others, because sometimes, no matter the work, it happens. But it has always been a point of growth—a point of relief—for both sides, whatever the outcome, when you can get things up and out. Some simply can't stand that kind of confrontation. That some endure is a true miracle and a gift above price. Linda and I are celebrating thirty years of friendship and we're still going strong.

I learned three things that day so long ago, and it stuck: (1) All relationships run amuck, they take airing and work. (2) The true ones endure because best truths are allowed and you just love each other. (3) "Best truth" spelled backwards is *"ouch!"*

I was just talking today with a close friend who feels she's lost someone. She's tried nicely a couple of times to get things sprouting again, but it seems to fizzle. I told her my Linda story.

"Bang on her door if you want her in your life," I counseled. "Tell her you love her, and miss her, and you're not giving up."

And don't.

Isabel Bearman Bucher

LIFE LESSON #2:
CULTIVATE INTIMACY

Many people skate along the surface of life, relating only on the most superficial of levels. We fail to experience the depth of connection that can only exist when we take the time and reveal the truth of who we are to another human being. The word intimacy is derived from the Latin *intimus,* which means innermost, deepest or most personal.

Have you ever noticed that you can begin a conversation with a friend feeling confused, then after she has truly listened to you, you not only feel reassured and relieved but you find that you can think more clearly? There's nothing more reassuring than being listened to. But this takes time. A steady diet of brief phone calls or hurried meetings just won't do. Your friendships need the luxury of a leisurely walk, a quiet dinner. They need space in which you can unwind and share.

> *Oh, the comfort, the inexpressible comfort of feeling safe with a person, having neither to weigh thoughts nor measure words, but pouring them all right out, just as they are . . .*
>
> *Dinah Maria Mulock Craik*

Everyone struggles to tend to friendships. You blame a

busy schedule; you forget about the value of those close to you; you take your friends for granted—it seems like too much trouble. And yet, you must put in the effort. While there are certain friendships that can survive a lack of interaction, most significant relationships require an investment of time, energy and attention. Regardless of where your friend lives, be it down the block or across the country, you have to make an effort to stay involved. Of course, there are those rare cases where months pass without your having spoken with a friend, and when you finally connect, it's as if no time has passed. But that's the exception. Most intimacy requires an ongoing dialogue. We're not suggesting that you have to talk with your friends on a daily basis, but on the other hand you can't allow too much time to pass without contact and expect to maintain a genuinely intimate friendship.

Authentic intimacy occurs in those connections with other people in which you can see and be seen, know and be known; in which you experience enough trust that you can reveal your innermost selves to one another. As you cultivate a greater level of intimacy in your relationships, your life will be enriched immeasurably.

I am taking the time to
nurture my significant relationships
and share my innermost thoughts,
feelings and dreams.

Knowing What Your Rope Is

Shortly after learning I had a rare type of breast cancer, one that would require a year of aggressive treatment, I decided to cut back on some of my activities.

I stopped by my son's classroom to explain to his teacher why I would no longer be coming to help every Monday morning. When I became upset as I told her about my diagnosis and the long months of treatment that lay ahead, she took both my hands, held them tightly, and told me this story about her friend Ann.

One summer, Ann decided to go river rafting. Everyone signed up for the trip had to learn the basic procedures and safety measures. As the instructor outlined the dangers, Ann became scared. What if her raft capsized or was dashed against the rocks? What if she were thrown into the rapidly churning water and carried downstream before anyone could rescue her?

The instructor had one answer to all of Ann's anxious questions: "There is a rope that is attached to the perimeter of the raft. Whatever happens, hold on to that rope. Never let go. Just hold on." And do you know what? An unexpected storm came up, and Ann's raft did capsize, but she remembered her instructor's words. She held on to that rope, and she survived.

I stared at my friend, wondering what this story had to do with me. "Know what your rope is, Myra," she counseled. "And hold on. Whatever it is. Through whatever happens. Just keep holding on."

She gave me a hug and returned to her classroom, leaving me to ponder her words. What was my rope? What would I hold on to in the days ahead? What would help me survive my perilous journey through the unknown world of chemotherapy, radiation and surgery? It didn't take me long to find the answer. My rope would be the love of my family and friends, who I knew would support me through whatever lay ahead.

As my treatment progressed, that rope was often at hand. It was there during my chemotherapy when my husband said, "Lean on me. I'll be here to give you strength. If you can't go on, I'll carry you until you're strong enough to continue on your own."

It was there the day of my surgery when a dear friend hung a silk carp, the Japanese symbol of courage, in my hospital room. It was there on Mother's Day when, unsure of what lay ahead, my daughter gave me an opal, the symbol of hope. And it was there one night after I had lost my hair, when I found fifty cents under my pillow with a note from the "hair fairy."

There were times during the year when I didn't get along with the people whose closeness and support I so desperately needed. I argued with my children about their refusal to attend a support group for families dealing with cancer. I fought with my husband over the handling of certain household matters.

In the past, I had been able to handle disagreements such as these easily, but at this particular time, I couldn't tolerate the feelings of loneliness and isolation that followed arguments. On these occasions, it felt as though the rope was slipping out of my hands and I feared the dark waters would engulf me. These were the most frightening days of all, because I knew I couldn't make it through a year of treatment alone. The love and laughter my family and friends gave me were just as essential to my survival as the chemotherapy and radiation treatments.

I discovered that Aristotle was right when he said, "Friendship is a thing most necessary to life, since without friends, no one would choose to live, though possessed of all other advantages."

And so throughout the entire year, I held on. I held on when it appeared as though my tumor wasn't shrinking as it was supposed to in response to the chemotherapy. I held on when a bone scan revealed a dark spot on a rib that looked suspiciously like bone cancer. I held on as though my life depended on it, because it *did.*

I survived my journey. My raft, although battered by storms and raging currents, is still afloat. I often hear my friend's words echoing in my mind: "Know what your rope is, Myra." I do, and I'm still holding on.

Myra Shostak

LIFE LESSON #3:
CHERISH YOUR FEMALE FRIENDS

"My women friends are my rock. They're lifesavers. I'd be lost without them." "My girlfriends keep me sane. I can talk with them about anything. I can call them anytime, day or night, and they'll be there."

These are some of the sentiments we have heard from women whether they are married, single, widowed or divorced. Friends, especially women friends, play an essential role in our lives. Men don't really leap at the chance to spend hours talking about their most intimate feelings.

Men tend to be problem solvers. They're generally more

comfortable with ideas and everyday, matter-of-fact situations. There is a depth of emotional intimacy that women experience with other women that rarely exists with men. Women love to explore their internal landscape—no schedule, no planned outcome—simply to listen and be listened to.

Many women find it easier to share the intricacies of their emotional lives with friends rather than with family members or with the person with whom they share a bed. While your spouse, children or family may have an investment in your remaining the same, your friends affirm and support your hopes and dreams. Your friends are a sounding board, they are a safe port in which you can explore your wildest, most outrageous thoughts and aspirations.

As you communicate the intricacies of your life to another person, you not only cultivate trust, but you come to know yourself in a new way. Your friends provide a new perspective on yourself and the world. Your women friends bring out different facets of your personality. They extend your thinking and expand who you are. As you share your struggles, insecurities, successes and joys, you begin to recognize that you are not alone. You are part of a larger community of women and this knowledge is incredibly comforting.

Your friendships can take many forms. Sometimes you mother one another. Sometimes you act as confidant and advisor. Sometimes you are the sister you always wished you'd had. And sometimes you're the perfect playmate.

The depth of my friendships depends,
in large measure, on how vulnerable I am willing
to be and how much of myself I share.

Basic Tool: Reconnecting

Choose five people you have depended upon when you've faced life's biggest challenges and experiences. These people are your anchors. Think of all the qualities, strengths and characteristics you appreciate about these people. For the next five days choose one person from your list and express your appreciation to him or her.

If acknowledging that person directly feels like too much, start by putting your thoughts in writing. Whatever you do, take the time to say thank you. Be sure to mention qualities you appreciate, special moments you've shared, and meaningful contributions this special person has made to your life. Tell him or her how their presence in your life has enriched you.

Another way of showing how much you appreciate someone is to practice random acts of kindness. Think of five caring things you could do for the people in your life that you love. Consider what each person enjoys, needs and cares about. These can be as simple as bringing a bouquet of flowers to a lunch date, picking your friend's kids up from school, filling up your husband's car with gas to save him time, shoveling the snow off your neighbor's walk, dropping off a pot of chicken soup to a friend who is feeling under the weather or making a donation to a charity in your friend's name. The possibilities are endless. Commit to doing five little things that remind the people you love how much they mean to you.

☕ Safety Pins and Postmen

The little things? The little moments?
They aren't little.

JON KABAT-ZINN

"What can I do to help?" Joel, my ten-year-old son asked. The shocking news of September 11, 2001, spread fast—even to ears thought too young to comprehend. But Joel did understand. He knew that his nation was wounded and that many lives had been changed forever. He understood that people were needing each other in a way that he had never seen before.

"But, really Mom, what can I do? What can I do to help the families, the kids and grown-ups?"

"Joel, you can pray. You know, praying is probably the most powerful thing you can do."

"Mom, I've already prayed, and more than one time a day! I want to know what *my hands* can do to help!"

I was now thinking on overload. I had no idea what a ten-year-old could do to help this situation, much less use his hands to do it with! I added to my prayer list, "An idea for Joel so that he can help victims of September 11th."

A day later, the thought came. "Joel, I've got it! Do you remember the beaded cross pin that you made at camp a couple of summers ago?"

"The one that was made of safety pins?"

"Yes! Why can't you try to design an American flag? You know, stringing red, white and blue beads onto safety pins. Then maybe you could collect donations to help the victims' families."

Off to the craft store we went, buying each and every pack of red, white and blue beads that we could find. Like on a scavenger hunt, we shopped for and bought safety pins. *Seventeen thousand* safety pins to be exact. Joel named his project "Helping Hands," and even found some friends who were willing to help assemble the flag pins. Joel then made signs that boldly read, "My Gift to You When You Donate to the Red Cross." Within weeks, Joel had managed to collect $5,000 in donations.

After such an overwhelming task, Joel's hands were tired. His fingers were tender. They had not yet recovered from accidental pokes from the sharp point of each safety pin, when he heard the horrific news—a postal worker had died from anthrax!

Again, the questions came flying. "Mom, what is anthrax? How did it get there? Aren't the postmen and women scared?"

I answered each question to the best of my knowledge.

But then came a question that I had no answer to, "Mom, what's the name of our postman?"

A lump formed in my throat as I realized that we had lived in our home for ten years, and I had no idea who had delivered our mail each day!

"Do you think our postman is scared?" Joel asked.

The next afternoon Joel stood next to our mailbox, singing to himself to pass the time until he saw the wheels of the U.S. mail truck. With a smile, he introduced himself to the mail carrier.

"Hi, I'm Joel. I live here."

"Glad to meet you, Joel. My name's Jimmy."

"Are ya scared?"

"Scared?"

"Yeah, about the anthrax."

"We're doing our jobs, and we're being extra careful. Thanks for asking," Jimmy said, just before he drove away.

I heard the door shut with gusto. "Mom!" Joel shouted. "His name is Jimmy! Our mailman's name is Jimmy!"

Within seconds, Joel met me in the kitchen. "I want to do more. Mom, I want to do something for Jimmy. Just how many friends at the post office do you think Jimmy has?"

"Maybe twenty?" I guessed as I got on the phone and called the post office. *Two hundred and five* was the count the postal worker gave. Evidently, Jimmy was both well-known and well-liked at the post office!

Again, Joel and I went to the craft stores to buy every red, white and blue bead we found. Due to their shortage of safety pins, we made calls, buying pins directly from the manufacturer. Joel rehung his sign, and "Helping Hands" was back in business.

This time it was different. Joel was not collecting donations. He was making gifts of encouragement—a flag pin for every postal worker in the city of Orange, California! After completing his task, Joel typed a note and printed it out two hundred and five times.

"I have made you this flag pin to remind you that people in our city appreciate the work you do for us. I am praying for you as you deliver our mail. I know that God will bless America! Love, Joel."

It was while Joel was attaching the notes to the flag pins that Allison, a neighbor friend, stopped by. "Hey, can I help?" she asked.

"Yeah. You've come just in time. I want to get these in the mailbox before the mailman comes!"

Joel quickly grabbed a pen, and Allison added her name to the notes. Sitting side-by-side, they worked until each flag pin was accompanied by a note. They then boxed up the couple hundred flag pins, tied a bow around them, and added a card that read, "To: Jimmy and Friends." They placed the package in our mailbox, and raised the red flag.

With a task well done, Joel and Allison went off to play.

It was not until later that afternoon that I got the call.

"Hi, are you Joel's mom?" the voice asked.

"Yes."

"Well, you must be very proud of your son. I am the postmaster in Orange, and I'd like to know if you would bring Joel and Allison to the post office tomorrow morning at about nine. I thought it would be great if they themselves could pass out the flag pins to the mail carriers."

The next morning came. The postmaster divided the 205 postal workers into three groups. Three times Joel and Allison took front stage encouraging the mail carriers and handing out pins.

Tears gathered in some of the postal workers' eyes as they received their pins from Joel and Allison. "I think it's fantastic that you two took the time to do this and come and talk to us," one man said while shaking Joel's hand. Others offered hugs and words of thanks. Before the morning was over, Joel and Allison were made honorary mail carriers of Orange, California.

Through this experience Joel has taught me many lessons. I've learned that the only requirements needed to help another are a set of "helping hands and a willing heart." Allison has reminded me that when my fingers are cracked and tender, it's time for me to call on a friend! Through the lives of two ten-years-olds, I am now assured that each of us can do something to help our nation heal.

From saying a prayer for those who pass you by to writing a letter to an unknown serviceman or stringing small beads, these gifts of time and love deeply affect those they touch.

"But, really Mom, what can *I* do? What can *my hands* do to help?" Joel asked.

I am proud of my son for doing something that never crossed my mind—for taking the time to care about others he had never met.

Janet Lynn Mitchell

LIFE LESSON #4:
SHOWER THE PEOPLE YOU LOVE WITH LOVE

It's easy to take for granted the people with whom you are the closest. You assume that they are mind readers and automatically know how much they mean to you and how much you care. Well, we hate to be the bearers of this harsh reality, but they don't. At least, you shouldn't assume that they do. You can't take your friendships for granted. Despite the fact that they'll rarely admit it, people crave acknowledgment. We all do. It's in great demand and short supply in our fast-paced culture.

What do we live for if not to make life less difficult for each other?

George Eliot

However, when you're traveling at the speed of light, you can miss this important detail. The solution is to slow down and recognize how much the people who support you mean to you. This includes everyone from your close friends to your children, your spouse or partner, the sales clerk at the video store, your mail carrier, your nanny and your children's teacher, as well as your family members. Just imagine how different the world would be if you took the time to extend these small kindnesses.

Take a moment and consider: When was the last time you acknowledged what someone important to you has contributed to your life? Have you told them how much you appreciate their thoughtfulness, their loyalty or their support? If you're like most of us, you're probably scrambling around in your mind trying to recall when you last shared your feelings of appreciation. The unfortunate truth is that we rarely do, especially not with those people with whom we are the closest.

You're probably pretty good at expressing your frustration, irritation

Questions Worth Asking

- Who brings joy and love into my life?
- Who makes me laugh?
- Which of my friends keeps me honest?
- Who encourages me to know the deeper truth about myself?

and dissatisfaction, but you need to get into the habit of speaking from your heart, and sharing your tender feelings. It may feel a bit awkward at first; however, when you express your appreciation, you not only strengthen the bond that exists between you, you set a precedent for future acknowledgments.

When you focus on all the support you have in your life, you realize how fortunate you are. As you become accustomed to expressing your appreciation, it will become second nature and will change the quality of your life.

I freely acknowledge and appreciate all the
people who support and encourage
the woman I am becoming.

☕ Ties That Bind

I had planned to take off work for a few days in order to tie up some loose ends.

What I hadn't planned was a new product launch two days before my wedding. Because I was the company's communications director, my presence was imperative. That's why my reception favors still weren't done when the wedding party arrived in town—at my house.

I'd only met my husband's family and friends once, and they'd never met my family. It was a chance for all to get acquainted before the big day. But there it all sat— deep-purple tulip bulbs, circles of tulle, satin ribbon and miniature acknowledgment cards—waiting to be assembled. I stared at the 150 sets trying to figure out how I'd ever find time before the wedding.

I calculated the evening hours ahead of me. If everyone left by 10:00 P.M., the project might take me until . . . oh . . . until about 3:00 A.M. Awful, I groaned, but manageable. I could do it.

During the evening, my guests noticed my tension and prodded me with questions, asking what they could do. Not the type to ask for assistance, I reluctantly admitted that I hadn't yet worked on the favors. They insisted on helping, despite my protests.

The women inspected the pieces of my project while I detailed how each bulb needed to be placed inside a foiled mini-cup, two layers of slippery tulle gathered around it, with a tiny thank-you note strung on a sliver of sleek ribbon to tie it off.

I hadn't predicted the dexterity required to do the job.

Over here a tulip popped out. Over there a bow slipped off. The tulle skewed. All thumbs, we were soon giggling like schoolgirls. And we erupted into full gales of laughter as we tried and tried again to tie our tulips. Finally, it dawned on us that if we teamed up as partners, one could hold the tulle while the other tied the tiny bow.

Aha. Now we were getting somewhere.

What would have taken me all night took only a couple of hours, even with the learning curve and joking that occurred. Of all the wedding favors assembled that night, the important ones were the new friendships we created.

We tied more than tulips. We tied families.

Pamela Gilchrist Corson

LIFE LESSON #5:
ASK FOR HELP

It's time for true confessions. When was the last time you asked anyone for anything—for help, for guidance, for directions, for information? Women are experts at finding resources for other people, but often struggle to ask for help for themselves. May we remind you once again that you don't have to do it all; in fact, you can't. More importantly, you have nothing to prove.

Women have been trained since birth that it's not polite to ask. It sounds ridiculous when you read it, but stop for a minute and see how you genuinely feel about asking. Most feel shy about considering their needs and stating them.

Part of the problem is that you're afraid you'll hear "no."

Ask, and it shall be given to you; seek, and ye shall find; knock, and it shall be opened unto you.

Matthew 7:7

This is understandable; no one likes rejection. However, too many women fall into the trap of thinking that if someone really cares about them, that special person should know what they need and provide it. No asking required.

Sounds great, but this kind of thinking won't get the job done. If you stubbornly wait for your friends and loved ones to read your mind, you're going to remain in a constant state of frustration, resentment and deprivation, which will ultimately leave you unsatisfied.

So, let us offer you an alternative to going it alone or waiting for your intimate circle to suddenly become psychic. Ask! That's the answer. It may feel scary, but you have to put yourself out there and start asking.

Ask your husband to take the kids to the park so you can have some time to yourself. Ask for a day off from work. Ask your children to clean up their toys. Ask the person sitting next to an open seat at the movies if they would move down so you and your friend can sit together. Ask your mother-in-law to bring her famous pot roast to Sunday dinner. Ask, ask, ask.

While there's no guarantee that other people will cooperate with your requests, at least you've put your wishes and desires out there for consideration. Ask for what you want and need. Ask clearly, politely and directly. You'll be amazed at how often you get a positive response. Ask for support. Ask for help. Ask for information. But whatever you do, begin to ask.

Questions Worth Asking

- What are three areas of my life where I could use help?
- What have I wanted to ask for help with, but haven't, either because I have been too shy or have just avoided asking?
- Who would be good resources to lend me support?
- When am I going to ask?

I easily and joyfully ask for what I need and want.

☕ The White Line

Sometimes an experience changes us forever. Life falls to the right or left of the white line it paints right down the center of your life.

When I was thirty-nine years old, my husband had a routine dye test to check his shortness of breath and stomach indigestion. No one could have possibly known how sick he was because he had just turned forty-two and was a young father of two daughters, five and nine. The test that day started a massive heart attack. I raced down a tiled hall beside his gurney shouting into his blue face to stay alive. He was sitting up, leaning on one elbow fighting for life and breath. Our hands broke apart as he disappeared with four doctors through double doors to emergency surgery. When those doors slammed shut, I experienced the loneliest, most bereft moment of my life.

LeRoy was a popular and well-known sports editor for our state's largest newspaper, so his condition was broadcast daily in all the media. Nobody knew from one minute to the next whether he'd make it through whatever day it was. I moved through those days in numb slow motion, trying to keep some semblance of order at home. I made the girls' lunches. I made the beds. I brushed my teeth. I took a bath . . . maybe.

I came and went to the hospital taking the seven flights of stairs to Intensive Care for exercise, but later I realized it was a kind of penance because he was so sick, and I was well. One day at a time. One foot in front of the other. One hundred forty steps. Sunrise. Sunset. The phone jangled, letters and cards poured in. People gathered at the hospital and at our home. Dreadfully weak, LeRoy continued having heart attacks after the nine-hour surgery. Most mornings, I'd find people on my doorstep, on the end of a phone or just sitting in my front yard or on my porch. The neighbors would come walking slowly down their drives and just raise a hand, or put it over their hearts. These gestures were the beginning of the painting job I came to call "The White Line," which would run smack down the center of my soul, my heart and my life. People asked what they could do to help, and, at first, I just mumbled this or that. One day, I returned to find the entire university football team in my backyard raking, clipping and bagging the fall debris. I vaguely remember telling Coach days before that my yard was a mess. The girls were picked up at school by an organized group of women who fed and bathed them, who sat through their homework, who went to school functions, because sometimes things were too bad to allow me to leave the hospital. How they knew, I never understood. One desolate, cold November night I returned home and found my next-door neighbor, Lorraine, sitting on the couch with our two mutt dogs in her lap.

"They're lonely," she said with a smile, while her hands patted the tops of both their heads. "Everybody always takes care of the girls but the dogs are left."

There was one horrible afternoon when LeRoy was so close to death I could barely breathe because I was now so tuned into his condition. In the midst of the collecting, growing and milling crowd, Sally, a tiny woman not taller than five feet, elbowed her way to the plastic hospital waiting room couch and sat beside me. She never said a word, and yet my world filled with her immense presence. Her clothes smelled line-dried and starched with just a vague scent of cinnamon graham crackers. She reached out with her eyes to mine, but it was her regular and quiet breathing onto which I was able to grasp. Breathing in and breathing out. In. Out. I went on that day on Sally's rising and falling chest. By sundown, LeRoy was rallying, yet another time. His doctors said he was fighting like a tiger with some inner something that was a pure miracle.

Nancy came daily and stitched an ABC border for her baby daughter's room. It collected and grew throughout the long days she kept me company—twenty-six individual letters became waxed with vines, strewn with flowers, enclosed in pale blue Xs. The pile of squares grew as the days passed. Somehow her stitching—dependable, patient, so forward-going—threw me a lifeline every time. I'd lost over twenty pounds because the thought of food made me sick. J.D. came bearing an enormous basket of fruit and placed a beautiful yellow pear into my hand. I stared down at it, and then, finding I wanted it more than anything in the world at that moment, I began to eat gustily, greedily. Its juice escaped from my mouth and dripped down my arm, trickling off my elbow. Never before, or since, have I tasted such a delicious thing. Next came, piece by piece, a beautiful orange, which he peeled, segmented and cleaned of veins with the care of a surgeon. He cracked nuts under his foot and picked the meats out carefully, offering them in almost perfect halves. He hand-fed me large russet grapes; his snowy, pressed handkerchief wiped my hands and face. Looking into his kind eyes, so obviously happy that his gift was so right, all of a sudden I laughed. Along with that fruit, which was then pumping nourishment into every capillary I had, his simple acts comforted me as surely as if I'd been lying in a cool river.

I couldn't, wouldn't, was absolutely afraid to cry because I thought if I did, somehow my tears would be throwing in the towel, signaling the death knell for LeRoy and my fortitude. Just what would the girls do if I fell down? In the middle of my street, I reported the day's latest to my neighbor. Alice's face had experienced the big bang, because freckles formed constellations all over it. Her great blue eyes filled, and I watched the water collect and run in streams down those stellar cheeks. Her simple tears washed some part of me that day because I was able to hug and try to comfort because she was so undone—I could fix Alice.

"I've come all dressed in red!" announced a teaching colleague, a few days later. She had arrived after I'd endured a particularly hard night at the hospital. Unable to find the energy to get dressed, I was wrapped in LeRoy's old blue terry robe and looked so terrible, she gasped, then held out her arms. I fell into those thin, old sticks, and she held me up as the tears that I had been desperately hanging on to broke the floodgates. They spilled off her narrow crimson shoulders and fell to the tile. Somehow that frail, willing shelf propped me up and oh my, I just let-'er-rip.

One evening close to Christmas, Toni, who sported a fat bottom lip, arrived at the hospital with candles, silver, china, a camouflaged bottle of sparkling white wine—her last, hoarded from a trip to Italy—and homemade minestrone. She'd pilfered one last rose from somebody's garden by sneaking over to the living room window and biting it off with her teeth. She'd called all the women in my life who now gathered round as she set a coffee table in the waiting room fit for a queen. Anybody on Albuquerque, New Mexico's Presbyterian Hospital Floor Seven who could be dragged out of bed that night by nurses, visiting family or bystanders, who pushed wheelchairs or propelled IV stands, paraded by our gathering, smiling, clapping and waving. Her act and our gathering lifted the spirits of the whole floor and mine too. Later we all got in a tight circle and sang "Home on the Range," of all things, which started a floor-wide song jubilee.

LeRoy never came home. His totally wrecked heart could not be fixed although he and his doctors fought a heroic battle. Two months after his surgery, he left this Earth at sundown, the first night of Hanukkah, December 18, 1976, speaking his last word, "Shalom," to his rabbi.

His bills soared to over $100,000 and our bank balance was exactly $84.32, because while LeRoy was a well-known journalist, his pay didn't match his renown. Months went by. The finances were worked out because by some miracle, the newspaper had instituted health and life insurance for its employees two weeks before his surgery. The deductible was written off by the hospital. I began the task of rebuilding our lives totally debt-free. Social Security widow's benefits allowed me to stay home with the girls.

It was a year before the humanity of that time began to reach me. During countless, grief-stricken nights, I sat up until the wee hours with my dogs on my lap sorting through the opaque, terrible hours of that time, able to listen only to Judy Collins songs. Then, something else began to reach me—faces, eyes, people started walking through the fog into my consciousness. I began to remember all their charity and their compassion—all their simple acts of mercy and of love. That's when the white line blazed true and fine before and straight through me.

It's been many years since LeRoy died. The girls have grown into beautiful, vital young women. I've remarried very happily. But one thing I know: In this world, good is stronger than evil, love is stronger than hate, and somewhere, somehow, like a beautiful flower, this magnificence of the individual human soul survives through the worst of times. Through wars, through terrible mayhem, it plants itself, grows and flowers again and again. It walks on through the smoke of sorrow and holds up a blazing brush full of white paint. I take everlasting comfort in that.

To all those who were with me during those awful hours . . . I return your kindnesses in moments of reflection and gratitude for my life and everything in it.

Thank you with all my heart. You changed my life and made me a painter, just like each of you.

Isabel Bearman Bucher

LIFE LESSON #6:
CREATE A CARING COMMUNITY

Community is defined as a body of people associated with a common pursuit. Community is an essential part of life. It gives your life meaning. Community makes you complete. It provides a sense of belonging. Community challenges you to be genuine, to share the deepest truths about yourself. It teaches you how to love and be loved, to care and be cared for. Community provides a safe harbor in the often stormy sea of life. A loving, supportive community is an essential ingredient for a rich, fulfilling life.

Your community can take many forms and have many layers of connection. You aren't going to share your innermost thoughts and feelings with each and every individual in your personal community, yet they are part of your support network nonetheless. Community exists in concentric circles beginning with those with whom you are most intimately connected, moving outward to include professional relationships, neighbors, coworkers, people with whom you share your faith, your nanny, the parents of your children's friends, teachers, etc.

Without a sense of caring, there can be no sense of community.

Anthony J. D'Angelo

Yet another layer encompasses your mail carrier, the check-out person at the grocery store, your doctor, dentist, massage therapist, personal trainer, hairdresser, accountant and your mechanic. All of these people, to a greater or lesser extent, are part of your larger community. Cherish them all.

*I am surrounding myself with loving,
caring people who support me in living
the life I am meant to live.*

Basic Tool: Your Support Team

Create a photo gallery or collage of the people who are your cheerleaders, your anchors, the people who lend you support and encouragement.

These can be family members, friends, coworkers, teachers, coaches or religious leaders. They can even be people you've never met, but who've inspired you, such as philosophers, poets, social activists, artists or athletes.

Along with a photo gallery, why not surround yourself with mementos supporting who you truly are, events that remind you of challenges you've met, goals achieved and experiences that have enriched your life? This is a way to remind yourself, especially during times of doubt, of all the resources that are at your disposal.

The Finishing Touch

WHAT IS THE STATE OF YOUR SUPPORT NETWORK?

Now that you've heard how important it is to have a solid support system, consider the extent and strength of your network.

Ask yourself, are there any holes in my extended support system?

If so, what can I do to begin to fill in the gaps?

Who, if anyone, is missing from my list?

Is there someone I've lost touch with, with whom I'd like to reconnect?

Who could I reach out to that I've never bothered to reach out to before?

What kinds of relationships would enhance my sense of community?

Once you've decided what is missing from your caring community, you can begin to attract kindred spirits. Use the Essential Ingredients you've learned, both here and in your life, to build the supportive community you need to realize your dreams and to live the life you deserve.

TAKE YOUR PASSION
AND MAKE IT HAPPEN

It is the soul's duty
to be loyal to its own desires.
It must abandon itself to
its master passion.

Rebecca West

Trooping with the Circus

Listen to the passion of your soul,
set the wings of your spirit free; and let
not a single song go unsung.

SYLVANA ROSSETTI

When I was five years old, I knew exactly what I wanted to do with my life. Every year my parents took me to the circus. I would sit entranced during the flying act. When it came time to leave, I felt the keen disappointment of merely watching from the sidelines. I dreamed of joining a flying trapeze act and trooping with the circus—quite a feat for a kid who wasn't lucky enough to grow up in a circus family and felt too shy to talk to strangers!

When I turned eight, my dreams were dashed when the ringmaster announced that the little boy performing in the flying act was six. I left that night practically in tears because I was already too old! Nevertheless, while growing up, I never outgrew my desire to "run away and join the circus."

Maybe wanderlust ran in my family. I remembered my father's marvelous stories about the days, long before my birth, when he'd traveled around the country booking his own shows. His passion: magic! I recalled browsing through his scrapbooks, reading neatly folded newspaper clippings from all over the country.

During my last year of college, a casual conversation fanned the flames of my childhood dream. It all started one hot August night when a woman on my skydiving team asked me if I would like to swing on the trapeze at the local YMCA. The first time I set foot in that gymnasium, a shiver of excitement made my breath catch in my throat. Spellbound, I watched as each flier climbed up, up and up higher still to a small wooden "pedestal," grabbed the "fly-bar," and sailed out over a huge net.

Weighing in at a trim 103 pounds, I easily scampered up the makeshift ladder. Once on the pedestal my confidence wavered, but an experienced flier stood behind me to help me off.

"I've got you," Manny said, putting one hand around my waist. "Reach out with both hands and grab the flybar when it swings towards you."

When the bar swung up, I released my death-grip on the side cables and curled my fingers around the white tape. Manny calmly lifted me up. I swung away from him, heart pounding, adrenaline pumping. After swinging back and forth four or five times, I let go and landed in the net. I was hooked!

When I eagerly told friends about this unique experience, they all asked the same question. "When are you going to run away and join the circus?" With a wistful sigh, my answer never varied: "I'm too old to do that." Even so, I lived for the nights when the fliers had use of the gym for two precious hours.

I met my future husband, Gary, in that gymnasium. Weeks later we talked to a man who had flown for Ringling Bros. We asked Bob if there was any way we could break into the circus as fliers. A couple weeks later, he whipped out a small spiral notebook and turned toward Gary. I leaned in.

"If you can learn all the tricks by Christmas," Bob said, "I can get both of you work for next season doing an act on my casting rig." A casting rig is a miniature, fourteen-foot-high self-supporting trapeze set up. Dumbstruck, Gary and I turned and stared at each other. Then, without a moment's hesitation, we both said, "Sure!"

We reached our goal by Christmas. Bob put in long hours that winter teaching us how to combine the hooks of the passing leap, and the various other tricks we'd learned, into the act that he and his ex-wife had done. Our daily practice sessions on the casting rig piqued the curiosity of Bob's next-door neighbor, Irene, and the three children she baby-sat. One week before we departed for our first show in Mesquite, Texas, Bob invited them over to see a dress rehearsal.

I watched them troop into the yard and plop down beside the rig, giggling. Our first audience! The true test had arrived. Would we rise to the challenge? Could we keep three toddlers entertained for seven entire minutes?

Gary and I donned brand-new costumes. The warm spring day yielded soothing sunshine and a light, cool breeze. While we warmed up, fluffy cotton-ball clouds started piling up for a flashy light show later.

We enjoyed playing to more than a silent yard full of overgrown weeds. Gary looked every bit the bumbling clown decked out in red polka-dot bloomers beneath baggy clown pants. When he took his first pratfall, the children's laughter distracted us so much that we almost forgot what came next! In our minds, we knew that the comedy should appeal to kids, but it took real children to plant that thought in our hearts. After my dismount, Gary pantomimed that he would catch me. But when he jumped into my arms instead, the kids couldn't stop laughing.

After we took our final bows, Gary flashed me a silly grin. We both knew that we had just taken the most challenging test we would face, and we had passed with flying clown clothes. Our toughest critics had laughed themselves silly. Look out Texas, here we come!

At our opening performance, I self-consciously peeked through the curtains from backstage, surveying the children in our audience. Even my butterflies had butterflies! Then I spotted a little girl who reminded me of Katy, one of the toddlers. Recalling the excitement we'd felt performing for the first time before those three kids, a light went on. I can do this!

"And now," Earl's voice boomed over the mike, "all the way from Denver, Colorado, prepare yourselves for rib-tickling antics on the low-flying trapeze with Grinn and Barrett!"

With that, we sailed out and began one of the most exciting careers of our lives. The act unfolded like clockwork. What beautiful, noisy children! By the time Gary's clown pants fell down revealing his matching turquoise costume beneath, the adults laughed out loud along with the kids. We finished to thunderous applause and breezed back through the curtains.

"We did it!" I said.

"What a great audience!" Gary added.

I glanced at the clock by the mall's glass elevator. "Just think, in two hours and forty-five minutes we get to do this all over again!" Thus began our life on the road trooping with TNT and Royal Olympic Circus—a small show that played inside shopping malls throughout the Midwest.

When I awoke the following morning, I exclaimed to

myself, "People aren't supposed to be this happy when they grow up, are they?" With a dazzling future beckoning to me, I eagerly slipped out of bed to embrace the new day.

Vickie Baker

LIFE LESSON #1:
DISCOVER YOUR AUTHENTIC PASSION

Authentic passion is the excitement you feel when you've discovered what you love. When you are passionately engaged, you are totally present. You are enlivened, focused. You lose sight of your surroundings, you forget yourself, your struggles, your day-to-day life. You're connected with something larger than yourself, something magical, something sacred.

You don't need endless time and perfect conditions. Do it now. Do it today. Do it for twenty minutes and watch your heart start beating.

Barbara Sher

An authentic passion can be anything from playing the piano, taking figure skating lessons, going antiquing, circulating a petition for a school bond initiative, creating a flower arrangement, trying a new gourmet recipe or taking a watercolor class, to volunteering to read to children at your local library. The possibilities are endless. It doesn't matter what you do as long as you take your passion and make it happen.

If you're going to create a life you love and live fully, you have to make passion your middle name. Authentic passion is time-released to consistently energize your life. It's a kind of passion that nourishes and sustains you—a passion that will feed your soul.

Authentic passion is becoming a regular part of my everyday life.

☕ Holding On to Dreams

Come to the edge, Life said.
They said: We are afraid.
Come to the edge, Life said.
They came. It pushed Them . . .
And They flew.

GUILLAUME APOLLINAIRE

Rain pounds against the classroom windows, and bursts of thunder boom from a layer of storm clouds. Pine trees lashed by the wind brush against the glass. If we were studying verbs and adjectives, my students' attention would be riveted on the stormy scene framed by the window. But it's indoor recess time, infinitely more exciting than grammar, and clumps of fifth-graders sit on the floor playing games, oblivious to the forces of nature and interested only in each other.

Standing at the board writing down a homework assignment, I hear snatches of conversation from a group of girls playing a game called Life. Their play has led to a discussion about what they want to be when they grow up. Blaine confidently announces she's going to be a dancer or a soft-ball player. "Softball's my first choice, though," she adds. Carolyn wants to train animals for movies, and Camille and Ashley are sure they'll be world-famous soccer stars. Ashley notices my feet standing on the hem of her skirt and asks, "Mrs. Ross, did you always want to be a teacher?"

I purposely drop the eraser and bend to pick it up, stalling for time while I think of an answer. Sometimes I feel like I was born a teacher. Especially when I go up in the attic and look in the dark corner where a mountain of boxes holds years of my life in the form of instructional materials for grade levels I used to teach.

Straightening up, eraser in hand, I respond, "Well, no. Actually I wanted to be an actress." This elicits giggles from eleven-year-olds that probably see me as a cross between their grandmothers and their daytime wardens, but it's a safe answer. After all, what eleven-year-old today doesn't envy the glamorous lives of actresses like Drew Barrymore, Cameron Diaz and Jennifer Lopez?

These girls would roar with laughter if they knew that at their age, I worshipped Mouseketeer Annette Funicello and longed to take her place kissing Frankie Avalon in front of rolling cameras on a beach party set.

Soon my students return to their game, and I climb over them to reach my desk and steal a few quiet minutes to remember. I feel a little guilty because I wasn't totally truthful. But how do you tell girls reared in a world of female professional athletes, politicians, astronauts and fighter pilots that their teacher's greatest aspiration for her future was to be the First Lady? And not any First Lady— but one just like Jacqueline Kennedy.

I remember being glued to the television to watch her 1962 tour of the restored White House and hanging on every word of her breathy voice flavored with that Boston accent. I examined newspapers, not for world affairs, but for pictures of her in French gowns, pastel suits, bright summer dresses, huge sunglasses and white pearls. I read of her triumphant tours of Europe where she bedazzled dignitaries with her graciousness, style and warmth, and the opulent state dinners she hosted in the White House. Everything in print about her became fodder for a scrapbook that grew to gigantic proportions.

Aspirations of achieving her elegance and charm inspired me to take a beauty workshop offered by *Seventeen* magazine where I desperately tried to walk balancing a book on my head and sit without crossing my legs at the knee. I took a foreign language in high school, not to achieve a graduation requirement, but to inspire awe and respect in preparation for my own future foray into politics as candidate for First Lady. Only, unlike my idol's beautiful command of French, I stumbled over the strange sounding words and verb conjugations, and failed the class miserably.

My scrapbook filled rapidly and spilled into a file folder stained with my tears when her husband died. No longer content to cut out pictures and articles, I saved entire sections of newspapers and magazines to remember those last dark days of a presidential reign the newspapers had started calling Camelot.

As I sit at my desk staring at rivulets of rain streaking the window, I realize I can't remember when I stopped adding to my scrapbook collection. Maybe it was when Jackie married her rich Greek and I thought she had deserted me. Or maybe it was my sophomore year in high school when a small part in "Cheaper by the Dozen" revived past yearnings for stage lights and acting glory.

A hungry student interrupts my thoughts to announce it's 12:30, which sends my fifth-graders clamoring to put away games and line up for the walk to the cafeteria. Thoughts of my future as First Lady are forgotten as we file out the door, hoping to beat fourth grade to the lunch line.

It isn't until later that evening when the dishes are done, and my husband who never had any aspirations of being president is watching TV, that I think again about my scrapbooks, file folders and dream to be the First Lady. It seems silly now. Why didn't I dream of being the President?

I think back to my fifth-graders playing Life and remember the enthusiasm in their voices when they spoke about their dreams for the future. Silly or not, dreams are important, I realize. Without them, little girls wouldn't grow up to be soccer stars, chemical engineers, dog trainers, actresses, even teachers. They wouldn't travel in space, defend our country in foreign lands or represent us in government.

As with all children who have ever dreamed, some will hold on to their dreams and make them come true, and some will not. But many of their dreams will change. Mine did. After I put away my scrapbook and my high school acting career fizzled, I found a new dream. I dreamed I'd be a teacher, just like my mother.

Suddenly I have a yearning to open that scrapbook, so I slip up the stairs and rummage in the storage closet. There behind a worn black cardboard hatbox bearing the pink logo of *Seventeen* magazine's Beauty Workshop, I see a storage box that I remember filling with albums and newspapers thirteen years ago when we moved into the house.

After prying open the lid, the first thing I see is Jacqueline Kennedy Onassis's dark eyes and soft smile staring up at me from the cover of the May 30, 1994 issue of *Newsweek*, the week after her death. Underneath it is my scrapbook. When I open it, transparent tape once binding articles and pictures to black pages falls in hard, rectangular clumps to my lap and brittle, yellowing newsprint slips to the center of the album.

As I pick through the piles, the words and images are

as clear as my memories of the youngster who dreamed of being Jacqueline Kennedy clad in a ball gown, sweeping down the White House staircase to greet her guests. And for just a moment I hear the rustle of satin and the faint strains of "Hail to the Chief."

Kris Hamm Ross

LIFE LESSON #2:
DREAM A LITTLE DREAM

Have you ever had the experience where you were involved in an activity, and time passed without your having noticed? Think back to the time before adolescence. What did you love to do? Was it riding horses? Was it taking acting or pottery classes? Did you love to play softball or climb trees? Were you a collector of coins, stamps or postcards from faraway places? Did you roller skate or ride bikes with your friends? What did you love to do?

You must go after your wish. As soon as you start to pursue a dream, your life wakes up and everything has meaning.

Barbara Sher

What happened to the passion you once felt? Where did it go? For many of you it was buried under the weight of

Questions Worth Asking

- What do I need to fan the flames of my passion?
- What can I do to make passion my middle name?

adolescence as you tried to fit into what was considered feminine. In order to be socially acceptable, many of you offered up your creativity, spontaneity, passion, enthusiasm and self-confidence to the god of conformity. In other words, you sacrificed yourself. Well now it's time to reclaim your passionate self and restore her to her rightful place in your life.

While each of you is going to redis-cover your passion in your own way, there is one thing you all have in common—your passion-ate self is just waiting to be invited back into your life.

*I embrace my passion
and it takes center stage in my life.*

Basic Tool: Your Nine-Year-Old Self

Let yourself drift back to when you were between the ages of seven and eleven, and recall the things you loved to do. List at least five activities you were passionate about. These should be five things that used to make time pass without you noticing it. These activities hold a clue as to what will feed your soul today. While your interests may be different now, what you were enthusiastic about in the past holds the germ of an idea for bringing passion back into your life.

☕ Leap into Life

One day, while sitting in a meeting with several male executives and watching them maneuver through a game of "one-upsmanship," a voice from within me whispered, "Run." I shook my head, trying to understand what had just happened. With sudden clarity, I realized I no longer wanted to be part of the high-stress, high-tech jungle of Silicon Valley.

I had just turned fifty. What did I want to do? I had no idea.

Later that month, I visited my mother in Idaho for a week of what she calls "hyacinths for the soul." She's always provided a loving, nonjudgmental environment where I could sort things out.

"I've never seen you so at odds with yourself," she said to me.

Mom was right. I'd always laid out my goals and marched forward, ticking them off as I passed by. I'd raised two children by myself. I'd progressed from secretary to vice president over the course of many careers. What I had figured out was that something was missing in my life. And I knew that doing more of what I was doing and getting more of what I was getting wasn't going to fill this unidentified void. I'd have to redefine "success" in some other way.

The last night in Boise, I had a dream. When I awoke, only one word remained in my consciousness. I looked it up in the dictionary: *enclave*—a minority culture group living within another culture. Having no idea how it could have meaning for me, I promptly forgot it.

Upon my return home, I found a complimentary edition of *International Living* in my stack of mail. The headline read: "Lake Chapala: An Enclave for American Retirees." Goosebumps crawled up my arms. I read further. A sidebar advertised a "Retire in Mexico" conference in Guadalajara the following month.

Enclave. I picked up the phone and made the reservation.

On my flight to Mexico, I sat next to an extraordinary Mexican woman. Brightly colored silk scarves draped around her body giving her a gypsy aura. Atop her graying auburn hair, Iona wore a huge chartreuse and white polka-dot bow. Daffodil earrings dangled above her fragile shoulders.

After we had talked awhile, Iona withdrew a velvet-wrapped package from her yellow straw bag. "Do you know this Tarot?" She asked, unwrapping a deck of oversized cards. "See how beautiful are the pictures."

I shook my head and smiled. "No, I'm afraid I'm not much of a believer in mystical phenomenon except for dreams."

Iona pulled down the food tray, swathed it with her burgundy velvet cloth and reverently set the cards on top. "Would you like that I am reading for you?"

Why not? What have I got to lose? I thought. "Will you tell me my future?"

"No. These cards are telling only what you know about yourself, but maybe are being afraid to see." Iona tipped her head slightly and peeked at me from the corner of her eye.

I nodded for her to continue.

"Bien, Karina, I am reading for you now from three cards only."

As instructed, I closed my eyes and concentrated on discovering what was missing in my life. I took a deep breath, shuffled the cards and placed them face down into three separate stacks.

Iona turned over the top card from each pile, caressing them with her milk glass fingers.

"Now, Karina, we begin. This card says who you are. The Fool, he means a new beginning or going into the unknown." Iona smiled at something she chose not to share with me and I wondered what new venture would greet me when we landed in Guadalajara. She continued. "When you are facing a difficult decision, the Fool, he tells you to follow your heart no matter how crazy it seems."

Maybe she could read my mind.

"Karina, you are The Fool." Her black eyes twinkled. "Such joy that is waiting for you."

I leaned back and closed my eyes. *She's just a little old lady with a bunch of cards,* I told myself. Then, unbidden from someplace deep within me, a little voice whispered, "Listen."

"This next card, The Hierophant, says that some things are getting in your way. They are keeping you from living the joyful life. This card says you are too much going along with what other people are expecting you to do maybe from churches or work."

Iona turned my chin toward her, forcing me to look into her deep mysterious eyes. "This was being comfortable for you, I think; but now is time for you to be not so comfortable and to be starting a new life, a life you live from here." Iona touched my heart. "And not from here," she said, tapping my forehead.

"Right now," I sighed, "I need to decide if I stay in my career or leave. It's scary. I know I've had enough of corporate America, but I don't know what else to do." I thought a minute. "I define myself by my job."

"*Si,*" Iona said, "this question is being the first step into your new life."

"And the last card?" I asked, with a pinch of sarcasm

and a dash of hope. "Will it tell me what to do next?"

"Let us see." Iona pressed the third card onto my palm. "Look. It is the Page of Wands." She cradled the back of my hand with hers. "Close now your eyes and pretend you are being at a train station." She spoke with a soothing, melodious voice. "A boy, he is holding out his hand to you from a train which is leaving. He smiles and yells, 'Jump! My train, it is going to marvelous places!' That boy, he is the Page of Wands." Iona paused, still holding my hand in hers. "Please to open your eyes now. The question is, Karina, are you jumping on that train and going with him?"

"It sounds tempting," I said, grinning. "But I have no idea where the train station is or where the train is going."

"These questions, they will soon be answered." Iona squeezed my hand. "Leap into this new life, Karina, and you will be finding your destiny."

That encounter with Iona occurred two years ago. Shortly after, I escaped the corporate rat race and moved to a wonderful cobblestoned village in Mexico. I left behind my spreadsheets and security, trusting that little voice within and those synchronistic signs planted in front of me to guide me along my way. I sold or gave away most of my possessions. My life is simpler now. It's balanced. It's happy.

I've identified that little voice inside me who begged me to listen. She is my little artist. She's been responsible for my writing and publishing a book, for my ventures into doll making, gourd crafting, pottery and painting. She's taught me to reprioritize my values, give back to the community and discover my own spirituality.

Living in the middle of Mexico without a watch, or panty hose or a cellular phone, and without the need to compete, succeed and acquire possessions, has freed me to reprioritize my values and to discover what was missing in my life. Wholeness.

Karen Blue

LIFE LESSON #3:
GO ON AN ADVENTURE

Countless women want to break the mold. They want to do something out of character. They want to have an experience that is going to change their lives. Do you ever feel like you'd like to do something out of the ordinary? Well stop wishing and start doing.

Where have you always dreamed of going? Is it hiking a section of the Appalachian Trail? Have you longed to

We cannot escape fear. We only transform it into a companion that accompanies us on all our exciting adventures . . . Take a risk a day—one small or bold stroke that will make you feel great once you have done it.

Susan Jeffers

visit Mt. Rushmore or tour New England to see the fall colors? Have you dreamed of snorkeling in the Great Barrier Reef or visiting Ireland to trace your family history? The destination is less important than doing something that will expand your sense of yourself. By going on an adventure, you allow yourself to step outside the well-worn paths of your everyday life; you expand your perspective and you enlarge your world.

What expeditions do you want to take? What adventures were abandoned either because of responsibilities or financial constraints? Is there someplace you've always dreamed of going, but never did? Do you want to tour the Inland Passage of Alaska? Have you always longed to lie on a beach in Hawaii? Did you want to hear a concert at the Grand Ole Opry or visit Graceland? These are pretty exotic escapades, but an adventure doesn't necessarily mean that you have to travel far from home or that you have to spend a lot of money. It simply requires that you do something out of the ordinary.

You can bring a sense of adventure into your life by doing something that isn't part of your everyday routine. You can become a tourist in your own town and visit places you've never been before. Spend your lunch hour exploring a thrift shop or browsing through a used bookstore. Take a bus to the nearest city and go to a museum or take a walking tour of the local cemetery. Explore parks or trails in your area. It doesn't take much to feel as if you've had a mini-vacation. Often it's as simple as interrupting your routine to experience a change of scenery.

I am doing something different,
something new, every day.

☕ The Birthday Tiara

*You will do foolish things, but
do them with enthusiasm.*

COLETTE

For my thirtieth birthday, I threw myself a soirée. My friend Sarah arrived early, sat me down and handed me a white cake box. A crown drawn in gold ink decorated the top. My heart leapt. After all, this was from Sarah, someone who gave the most meaningful gifts.

I peeled back the lid. Nestled amidst star-splattered tissue paper was my very own crown. Brightly colored candles sprouted from a framework of iridescent pipe cleaners.

"It's a birthday tiara," said Sarah. "And you have to wear it."

I laughed. She knew I needed permission.

And so, for one night, I felt like a celebrity surrounded by adoring fans. But after the festivities, I packed up my treasure and stowed it away. I'd had my night of stardom.

A few years later, I remembered my tiara. I decided to

display it amidst the children's books in my study. Glancing up from my computer, I'd notice it and smile.

Then came another birthday. My thirty-fourth. They were all beginning to feel the same. After I opened my gifts from my husband John, I told myself, *This will be a nice day.*

I said my morning prayers. Sitting up from where I had reclined on the rug I spied the crown. *Should I?* I thought. *No. That's silly.*

But then I heard a louder voice. *John's gone to work . . . I'm home alone . . . Why not?*

I plunked it on my head. Chuckling, I smiled ear to ear. I felt lighthearted as I got ready for work, like I'd been zapped with a tiny current of energy and joy. Was that me twirling around the kitchen?

Singing goodbye to the kitties, I grabbed my car keys and purse. Then a voice in my head yelled, *Stop! You're not wearing that out, are you?*

I froze. What would people think? I must be nuts.

But wait, said the new, fun-loving me. *It'll be an experiment. Let's see how many motorists notice.*

I was bitterly disappointed when not a soul looked my way during my commute. *Now what?* I thought, sitting in the parking lot at work. *Do I wear it in?*

Stares of disbelief greeted me at the museum staff entrance. The security supervisor trailed me, a grin on his face. He pummeled me with questions like, "What is that thing? Does it light up? How old are you?" I answered the first two, and ignored the third.

My female colleagues embraced my new look. "I love it," they exclaimed, showering me with accolades. "You have to wear it for your school group."

I met the fourth-graders from Fairfax and immediately addressed a few open mouths and wide eyes. "Does anyone know why I'm wearing this?"

A hand shot up. "You wanna look silly?" blurted out a youngster.

A chorus of giggles met my feigned hurt look.

Another student, as if to make amends for his rude classmate, asked if they could sing "Happy Birthday" to me.

"At the end of the tour," I promised, tickled.

Walking next door to meet my friend Brittney for lunch, I thought about my headpiece. It's really like a hat, I rationalized. Hey! I can wear those now! I'd always been envious of the stylish creations worn by older women at church.

I shared with Brittney what I'd observed so far. "Women congratulate me. I think they all secretly long to wear one. Children stare or ignore it. They're the most polite. Men try and guess my age, then ask, 'Does it light up?' I'm getting sick of that one. Guys and their toys!"

"It's lit from within," said Brittney. Girls are so gushy.

My tiara slipped off that afternoon. I insisted my stylist wear it while she cut my hair.

"You don't need it, Miriam," teased her boss. "You already think you're a queen."

By the time I drove to meet my husband at his office, I'd practically forgotten what was on my head. But he noticed.

"You've worn that all day?" he asked in disbelief.

"Yup," I replied. "And I'm not taking it off now."

He threatened to bail out on our evening together, but I was armed. "It's my birthday. One day out of 365."

He knew he was beat.

At the restaurant I was greeted with the typical responses I'd heard all day. Except for one. En route to the restroom, a very vocal woman shouted at me, "When you gonna light your candles?"

"I can't," I told her, amused. "They're plastic." Her face fell in disappointment.

It was after midnight when I finally returned my tiara to its spot on the bookcase. Another birthday had come and gone. But a very different one. Why? Because I had made it so. I had risked. Tiptoeing at first, tempted to turn back, I had ventured beyond the safe and secure. I'd found courage within myself. As one friend remarked, I was "gutsy and glorious." And this was only the start.

Deborah M. Ritz

LIFE LESSON #4:
BE OUTRAGEOUS

It's time to be outrageous. What do you have to lose? You don't have to impress anyone. It's time to please yourself, to celebrate who you are and to be uninhibitedly yourself.

Buy a jar of bubbles and at a stoplight spread bubbles for the passersby. Wave at people you don't know. Send yourself a bouquet of balloons that reads "Congratulations!" and simply celebrate the fact that you're you. Make mud pies or go to the beach and make a sand castle. Meet a friend for dinner and wear a pair of wax lips. Buy yourself some yummy new sheets that make you feel either cozy and comfy or sexy and alluring. The choice is yours, just make it something that borders on the outrageous.

Mix a little foolishness with your prudence: It's good to be silly at the right moment.

Horace

Try something you haven't done before. If you've never been athletic, why not take a tai chi class or learn karate? If you've always felt that you don't have an artistic bone in your body, sign up for a painting class, or a weekend welding workshop for women. If you've had the same haircut for years, why not get a makeover and change your style completely? If your house is painted tastefully beige—or tastefully any color—spice things up with a splash of color. If you've always admired people who are outspoken and express their political views, but never felt the moment was right to speak up yourself, now is the time to volunteer on a campaign or go on a protest march. Forget being prudent, sensible, appropriate and grown-up for a moment and do something outrageous!

I take risks that bring me to the edge of myself and cause me to grow.

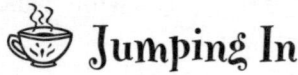 Jumping In

Play is the exultation of the possible.

MARTIN BUBER

The worst thing about growing up is the ease with which we surrender ourselves to the details of daily living. One autumn the leaves were particularly glorious, the color of Halloween pumpkins and childhood sunsets. But driving through the country to work I noticed the gaudy colors only in passing. Instead, I obsessed about nits: picking up children from school, the latest deadline at work, or household chores and projects. The colors passed without my noticing.

Until, one day, my four-year-old, with the wonder Columbus must have felt upon gaping at the New World, contemplated the small mountain of leaves her father had raked, turned to me and said, "Let's jump in."

I can't take credit for her understanding, correctly, that one autumn leaf is to be admired, but more than several dozen are meant to be plowed into. That knowledge was instinctive on her part, as it is for anyone under three feet tall.

I certainly set no happy-go-lucky example for her. I

hadn't tumbled in leaves for more than twenty years. Worse, when my daughter gazed upon the mound, I was standing in the driveway with briefcase in one hand, car keys in the other, high heels, business suit and what was probably a horrified expression on my face.

You don't get it, I explained in so many words. It's your job to jump in leaves. You're the little kid here. I'm the grownup, dull, predictable, and utterly incapable of doing anything so senseless, unreasoning and delightful. Why can't you jump in the pile alone?

"Please," she said.

My clothes, I said. Children's clothes are made for jumping in leaves. Not those of adults. I'd get a run in my stocking. I might get my suit dirty and have to get it dry-cleaned. Even if I didn't, I pictured myself pulling out a crumpled, dry leaf from my pocket in the middle of a business meeting.

"Please, Mom," she said, gazing up at me with her coal-dark eyes.

"Okay," I relented.

That is how I discovered the joy of diving in a small mountain of leaves, high heels first, business suit akimbo, clutching the guiding hand of my small daughter.

Anna was right. Although she didn't understand or artic-ulate her reluctance to wait for me while I got changed into my jeans before I jumped, I knew afterward that it would have been all wrong. Diving into leaves isn't a big deal. But there is something about jumping in leaves and not caring about suit, shirt or dignity that makes the experience wonderful. Like splashing in a puddle on purpose, or trying to catch snowflakes with your tongue. It is not so much an act as a state of mind; of being willing to wear the world lightly, if only for a few minutes. Years later, my son Tim taught me the same lesson all over again when he showed the same joy of jumping in leaves.

The view from the leaf pile helps you notice things that are easy to overlook: the china-bowl blue sky, how beautiful is the short pause of autumn before cold begins in earnest. Not to mention how much fun it is to bury yourself in leaves up to your neck.

While that long-ago fall with Anna lasted, every day she and I joined hands and, after building momentum by running down the driveway, we jumped in leaves.

The memory has made me think: Maybe this winter, I'll make angels in the snow.

Maura J. Casey

LIFE LESSON #5:
LIVE YOUR PASSION

You probably have secret wishes and desires that you've buried under the needs of children, families, work—things you've been meaning to do, but haven't gotten around to doing. It's all too easy to abandon your dreams in the face of your busy life. But, when you neglect your dreams, your life becomes a bit blander and more lackluster. Unfortunately, you do as well.

Each of us has a fire in our heart for something. It's our goal in life to find it and to keep it lit.

Mary Lou Retton

A passion isn't a gentle need; it's a craving. Those of you who were once pregnant will remember the power of cravings. While we're not talking about food here, the necessity is exactly the same. Your passion is what you are the most deeply curious about, what you hunger for. It's what you would do even if no one ever saw or acknowledged your efforts. Your passion is what you would do if you stopped worrying about pleasing anyone but yourself. It's the most urgent wish that is being whispered by your heart. Your passion is what you long to do in the deepest recesses of your being. It is what will electrify and enliven your life.

And the day came when the risk to remain tight in a bud was more painful than the risk it took to blossom.

Anaïs Nin

Take a moment and think about what your dream was before it was buried under the weight of your everyday life. What do you truly love? If money wasn't an issue, what would you do? Just allow yourself to dream. You're under no obligation to do any of the things that pop into your mind. So relax and just let your imagination run free.

Why not write down your secret wishes and desires? Don't censor yourself. You don't have to show them to anyone. They are just for you. These dreams are your inspiration. They can become a blueprint for rediscovering your passionate self.

Once you've written down your secret wishes and desires, pick one—when you see the list you'll know in your heart which one you truly want to pursue first—and do something to make that dream a reality by the end of the month. Any action you take will give you an instant infusion of energy and begin to revive your passion.

I am reconnecting with my passionate self and discovering greater self-expression and creativity.

Basic Tool: Create a Passion Kit

To start, find the perfect box or container. This is important. Choose exactly what you want to hold the ingredients that can bring a sense of joy, creativity and playfulness back into your life.

Now ask yourself: What do I need to rekindle the passion in my life? Is it a new pair of pinking shears, a set of watercolors, a sheaf of sheet music, a basket of gardening tools, a packet of travel brochures? Whatever it is, get it. Indulge yourself.

Here are just a few examples of what women have done to rediscover their passion. One woman who had abandoned her love of horseback riding when she entered adolescence, included a booklet of horse stickers to symbolically represent her rediscovered passion. She then went on to buy a pair of jodhpurs and boots, and began taking riding lessons. Another woman who had loved to sew, but no longer had the time to indulge this interest, started to collect fabric for a crazy quilt she had always wanted to make. She dug her sewing machine out of the attic and joined a quilting club. Yet another woman remembered taking pottery classes as a girl. She put a small ceramic figurine in her passion kit. Soon her recollection had rekindled such joy that she bought a bag of clay, set up a wheel in her basement and began to make pots. She rented space in a kiln to fire her creations and eventually took classes in ceramics.

You know how excited children get when you take them to a toy store? Well, that's the feeling you should have when you think about stocking your passion kit. It's time to indulge your heart's desire. Get your creative juices flowing. While your budget may not permit you to buy *all* of the necessary ingredients at one time, you can make a start.

The Finishing Touch

WHAT HAVE YOU ALWAYS WANTED TO DO?

It's time to get out a piece of paper—or better yet, your journal—and create a Dream History. This is a record of all the different forms your passion has taken throughout your life. Start at the beginning and work forward. Here is an example:

At 7 . . . I dreamed of riding horses

At 12 . . . I dreamed of becoming an actress

At 17 . . . I dreamed of going away to college and meeting new friends

At 20 . . . I dreamed of being a documentary filmmaker

At 25 . . . I dreamed of moving to Mexico City

At 30 . . .

At 40 . . .

Look over your list and add places you wanted to go, goals you wanted to accomplish, lifestyles you longed for, things you wanted to try.

Now make your current Dream List. Start with today and make a similar list of your dreams and desires for this month, this year, three years from now, five years from now. Complete the following statements for each entry: "I want ___", "I need ___", "I dream ___". And don't forget to be as specific as possible. That's how you take your passion and make it happen.

Essential Ingredient 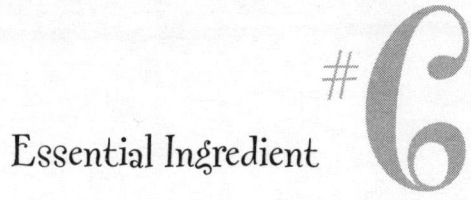 # 6

MAKE EVERY DAY SACRED

The great essential ingredient . . . is that the
sacred is in the ordinary, that it is to
be found in one's daily life.

Abraham Maslow

☕ Daydreams Die

In my history, there is a certain moment in time that, if I could, I would build a monument to its memory.

One sunny afternoon, while driving down a country highway and enviously admiring the lovely homes in their idyllic settings, I allowed soft rock music to lure me down into my pond of daydreams.

Daydreams were a way of life for me back then, an escape from the mundane life I led as a wife, mother and full-time nurse. Eternal struggles to provide just the basics—rent, food, new sneakers for the kids—wearied me. Surrounded by epicurean friends and neighbors, I had developed a lust for all things material. Often frustrated, I spent many waking hours afloat in my lagoon of wishes, enjoying the illusion of wealth, fame and leisure—my daydream destiny.

Lately, this hidden lagoon had begun to metamorphose into a swamp, a murky sludge where I'd plot and scheme to manipulate myself out of the relationships that held me back from a life of sophistication, adventure and pleasure. Darker dreams held more perverse options.

Suddenly I surfaced back to reality and the highway.

The big semi-truck up ahead unexpectedly veered to the right. I watched in curiosity as a red Yugo flew upward over the truck and passed by the side of my station wagon. The little car arced downward and the driver glanced at me. No fear did I see, only bewilderment. Before I could blink, the front of his car nosed into the highway with a dull clunk, rear wheels spinning at the sky. It remained that way, like an ostrich buried in the sand. As I ran toward the site, there was silence. No birds sang, no people called out. The world paused in attention.

His left arm hung out the open window. A small trickle of blood appeared from under the sleeve of his crisp white shirt. The steering wheel was embedded in his face, just under his nose, and the engine sat in his lap, hiding his lower body. I felt for a pulse. At that moment, the man lifted his head and took a deep, shuddering breath. He looked me straight in the eye. Somehow, despite the utter destruction of his lower face, he managed to murmur, "Tell them I love. . . ," and then he died. I held his hand and prayed the Prayer for the Dead. When I opened my eyes, the world woke up again. I became conscious of a small, respectful crowd gathered nearby, heads bowed and holding hands in companionable prayer.

The ambulance arrived and I left the scene, knowing Mr. George Brown wasn't there any longer. As I drove away, I was overcome with the momentous changes that had just occurred in so many lives. In seconds, the lives of his children, his wife and his friends had been forever altered. Was he rich, was he poor—was he revered or reviled? Did it matter anymore?

Stunned by my reaction to this abrupt death, and heartened by the connectedness of that silent crowd, I shed a few shocked tears. I knew that this was a life-changing moment. Wants fade to insignificance in light of our ultimate destiny. An unknown and quiet peace—a sense of inner joy and sincere appreciation for life—entered my heart that day.

An unknown man's final thoughts were not of riches or fame, but of the people he loved. His words became a candle in the dark just for me . . . to illuminate a path of understanding and love and to kill daydreams born of fruitless frustration and needless regret.

Lynne Zielinski

LIFE LESSON #1:
REMEMBER WHAT'S IMPORTANT

Sometimes, despite your success in the world, you may feel that there has to be more to life—you may feel a longing for a connection with "something" that you can't quite put into words, but that you know you've been missing. You may feel a hunger to go deeper in your life, to move beyond the outer trappings of the world, so you can connect with something larger than yourself.

There's nothing wrong with wanting fine china, a pair of diamond earrings or a cashmere sweater. It's just that in our culture things have gotten way out of balance. Our desire to have more is continually being stimulated by the media. We're bombarded with commercials, movies, billboards and magazines filled with beautiful people, extravagant homes, cars, clothes and jewelry—you name it.

Unfortunately, in our consumer-driven culture, it's easy to lose sight of what's truly important. You desire deeper meaning in your life, but do you really think that hunger can be fulfilled by a new car, an all-expenses-paid shopping spree at your favorite clothing store or a trip to the plastic surgeon? Probably not. However, advertisers continually try to sell you what you don't need. And unfortunately, you believe them.

The question is, how can you find your fulfillment in

something that goes beyond the trappings of everyday life? Sure, this is a challenge, especially in our materialistic society, but it is possible for you to make every day sacred.

I am finding deeper meaning in my life.

☕ Who Wants to Be a Millionaire Anyway?

There are two ways to be rich;
one is to have more, the other is to want less.

DICK LEIDER

I was okay with seeing the picture of the newest game show millionaire on the cover of that magazine. Really, I was. After all, it's no small achievement to know that there are seven countries in Central America, that tapioca comes from the cassava plant, and that the Artist Formerly Known as Prince was formerly known as Roger Nelson. Good for you, Mr. Millionaire Who as of Last Week Was Still Driving a Dodge Dart. I'm happy for you, your adoring wife, and those two kids of yours who are now secure in the knowledge that their overbites can, and will, be corrected.

The story about the woman on the East Coast who won a gazillion dollars in the lottery a few months ago didn't bother me all that much either. She seemed so nice. So worthy. Especially when she said she was going to use the money to end hunger in her favorite Third World country, shortly after her spree at Bloomingdale's.

And I had no problem with the lady who won that huge slot-machine jackpot. Or all those twenty-year-old barefoot billionaires and their garage-based computer businesses. Maybe those guys will have time now to buy socks and some pants that fit right.

When it comes to other people's fortunes, I think I have, for the most part, been downright magnanimous. But there's only so much we hard-working non-millionaires can take. And with recent news from the stock market, I may have reached my limit.

First, a little background. At the beginning of last year, I came into an unexpected inheritance from a long-lost aunt. Not enough to buy a Tuscan villa or even a new Toyota, but enough to make me think that perhaps I, too, should hop aboard America's Investment Express.

So I consulted a highly regarded financial planner who, by the way, had an excellent haircut, a fresh manicure and enough Italian marble in his lobby to dispel any doubts about his abilities. He asked about my "tolerance for risk." When I said "moderate," he recommended certain mutual funds with a "proven track record"—funds he said he'd be willing to put his own money into, if his portfolio weren't already so darn diversified. He spoke of those who managed these accounts—the folks smiling there in the annual reports fanning across the gleaming football-field expanse of his rosewood desk—as if he personally knew their shoe sizes and the names of their children.

"So, want to move ahead on this?" he called over from his swiveling, all-leather chair with lumbar support, sliding a weighty pen in the direction of my checkbook.

But I barely heard him. In my mind I was far, far away—in that land where people live off their interest.

Before the quarterly reports started arriving in the mail, the thought had never crossed my mind that investments could actually lose money. I blithely believed it was simply a question of double- versus triple-digit growth.

Wrong. At a time when headlines ecstatically proclaimed news of bull markets and an investors' heyday, my money was busy packing its bags and heading south. Seems the managers of my particular funds, hedging their bets about the American economy, had boldly ventured into a variety of foreign markets. So while NASDAQ was setting new records, my little nest egg was, apparently, helping to support ventures like fisheries in the Ganges and accordion start-ups in Warsaw.

"Well, live and learn," I gulped after the third consecutive quarter of double-digit losses, adding with just the slightest hint of sob, "Hey, it's only money."

Then along comes the incredible stock-market success of the San Diego-based high-tech company known as Qualcomm.

I know lots of people who work there. People who through the years took advantage of all their stock options. They're the same friends I've bumped into waiting for mini-quiche samples at Costco. Neighbors who've phoned to ask, "Do you by any chance still have that section of the newspaper with the 40 percent off coupon from Mervyn's?" People who at this very moment are watching their new big screen TVs, debating whether to add on or move up, and planning their Easter-week cruises for the whole family, plus Grandma.

So I do the math. I calculate what my earnings would have been if, instead of funding all those Yak Breeders with Big Ideas, I had put my money into that local stock at the beginning of last year. Alas, the display on my handheld calculator isn't big enough to accommodate a number with so many zeros.

But when I finally pick myself up off the floor, I begin to see things more clearly. Does wealth really matter? I ask myself. Would the colors of a sunset be more beautiful with a bigger bank balance? A full moon any fuller? A child's smile or a lover's touch any sweeter? With a cool million or two available at the ATM, would that morning cup of French roast taste any richer? Would the sight of a good friend's face be more welcome? And what about the pleasures of a walk on the beach? Would the crashing waves be more dramatic? The pelicans sillier-looking? The sun on my shoulders warmer? I ponder these questions, all the while enjoying good health in a fine city and a favorite song on the radio.

No, I decide. Definitely not. Riches have little to do with real contentment.

And yes, Regis, that is my final answer.

Sue Diaz

Life Lesson #2:
Embrace Simplicity

The truth is, most of us have too much—we have too many possessions, too much food, too many places to go, too many choices. When you stop and think about it, this is the first time in history that we've been faced with this problem—the problem of having too much. In fact, many of us are exhausting ourselves in the pursuit of having it all.

Simplify, simplify, simplify.
Henry David Thoreau

To what extent is desire running your life? We all get caught up, to some degree, in the desire to have it all. We think that having a new car, living in a certain neighborhood, having just the right wardrobe will bring us happiness. But very few of us experience the life we see on

TV. Ads suggest that if you just had the right makeup and the newest fashions, your life would be great. However, most of us don't find this to be true.

Live simply so that others may simply live.

Gandhi

You have to come to terms with the reality that you can't have everything you want. You may want a new car with air conditioning and a video player for the kids, but what you need is safe, reliable transportation. You may want a new house with more bedrooms and a pool, but what you need is shelter: comfortable surroundings in a safe neighborhood. You may want a new wardrobe, but what you need are serviceable, attractive clothes that will suit your various activities.

In order to live a quality life, you need to distinguish between your wants and your needs. Needs are these things essential to your survival and growth. For example, food, shelter, water and clothing all qualify as needs. Wants are the extras—the things that satisfy your desires.

Food for Thought

Instead of thinking about the person who has more than you, spend your time thinking about those who have less. It will make you more grateful—and hopefully more giving.

We're not suggesting you move to a cabin in the woods and sell all your worldly possessions, grow your own food and make your own clothes. We are recommending that you figure out how to simplify your life right where you are.

- Do I have everything I need right now?
- Has my lifestyle become more important than my life?
- What does simplifying mean to me?
- What benefits would I reap from living more simply?

Simplicity is about reducing the things in your life that no longer serve you, eliminating energy-draining activities, and most of all, adjusting your attitude.

Simplicity is extremely personal. What may be simple for someone else may not be simple for you. While one person may consider their cell phone to be a tool that simplifies life, another might decide that it's an annoyance that needs to go. There is no rule for how many changes of clothes you should have in your closet or whether you should own a DVD or keep the vase your Great-Aunt Selma gave you. It's all about stripping back the possessions, activities and habits that eat up your time and energy so that you can focus on what truly matters.

Having either too much or too little diminishes the capacity to live life to its fullest. It's only when you know the difference between what you want and what you need that you can begin to pare down the excess and find a middle ground. Through simplicity, you discover the ways in which consumption, activity, possessions and habits obstruct your life.

Simplicity is the freedom from mental and emotional

clutter. There are no rules, no blueprints, no external measurements of how simplicity works in your life. It's up to you to determine whether what you have and what you do enhances or impedes what's truly meaningful.

With simplicity, your life becomes clearer, less complicated, more direct and less ostentatious. As you simplify your life, you'll experience more inner peace, a more conscious use of your time, less clutter, fewer involvements and more orderly routines.

Choose simplicity in small ways. Just take one step in the direction of simplification, be it calling a moratorium on shopping, declining a dinner date, cutting back on your children's after-school activities, or cleaning out your closet. It's a demanding discipline, but well worth the effort. Simplifying your life is a process that takes time. After all, it took years for your life to become complicated, and it's not going to be reversed in a day or a week.

I am simplifying my life and enjoying the benefits of more time and greater inner peace.

Basic Tool: A Buyer's Quiz

Before you buy something, ask yourself the following questions:

Do I really need it?
How often am I going to use it?
Where will I put it?
Is this something that will truly enhance my life?

A Quiet Place

I found a quiet place today in the hustle and bustle of my life. I didn't think to go searching there, and really, I didn't find it, it found me. All this time this quiet place I longed for was within me.

I was sitting with my feet up on the coffee table in front of a roaring fire on a cold and windy afternoon with my two-month-old daughter snuggled up close to my breast, asleep in my arms. My three-year-old daughter lay asleep beside us, with her bottle of chocolate milk still in her grip, but lying on its side dripping slow drips of chocolate milk off the side of the couch. Our puppy was curled up in a corner sound asleep. I could hear the little in-and-out roars of his puppy snores. Finally, a quiet place I could go to put my feet up and relax, to make decisions, plan vacations, enjoy the new paint color of the living room, reflect on mistakes, smile over triumphs and give thanks to God for the many miracles I've witnessed thus far in my life.

It dawned on me during this moment of bliss that my life is exactly what I wanted it to be. Oh sure, I had many dreams as a child, ambitions and goals that I set and lived by. I wanted to be a *teacher,* a *writer* and a *dancer.* And although I wouldn't say it out loud, I really, really wanted to be a mom. And not just any ol' mom. I wanted to be the mom all the kids in the neighborhood knew and liked and called by her first name. I wanted to be the kind of mom that didn't mind if her daughter ran through the sprinklers fully dressed on a hot summer afternoon, just because. I wanted to stop my career in full swing to stay home with my kids and witness all the marvels of their world at their moment of discovery. I envisioned reading Dr. Seuss and Amelia Bedelia books to them as we sat close together on the couch under blankets, sipping hot cocoa. I longed to share with them my mistakes and shortcomings, so they wouldn't feel less than they are, or feel they had to be perfect. I saw myself screaming, "Great job!" on the sidelines of soccer games, dance recitals and spelling bees. I pictured a lot of hugs and kisses and a lot of "I love yous" for no reason at all, several times a day. I didn't realize that becoming a mom would allow me to be all these things and so much more.

As a *teacher*, teaching my daughters to embrace the beautiful people they are and the women they will become is a gift and a blessing beyond words. Teaching them about life, the world, our family, values, love, music, sunsets, puppy licks, why snowflakes disappear, about self-esteem, self-respect, dreams and disappointments, fills me with a sense of purpose, meaning and love that no position or salary could eclipse.

As a *writer*, my daughters inspire me to dig deep down into the trenches of my own childhood, take notice of the silver linings of my heart and stretch to the far reaches of my mind to express what my soul truly cannot contain. To my surprise, I have written so much more as a mother, than before I had children in my life. I have been inspired to write about things closest to my heart, which always produces better writing. I have even had several short stories published, in hopes of inspiring someone else by sharing my experiences (both good and bad), as a mother, a daughter and a woman.

My oldest daughter Jessica also loves to dance. She is three years old. So, every chance we get, we turn on the CD player in the kitchen while we are baking cookies, eating lunch or emptying the dishwasher and we get all sweaty dancing to old school hits and a few current ones too. Right now, our favorite song is "The Game of Love" by Carlos Santana and Michelle Branch.

To some, my life may seem simple, but to me, it is far richer than I ever imagined it could be. If twenty years ago I was asked to describe what I thought would be the ideal life, I know it wouldn't be what my life is today.

What makes it so wonderful? Having a fire every night during winter, playing Candyland, Play-Doh and writing with chalk on the sidewalk. Hearing my husband getting ready for work in the morning, his gentle kiss on my cheek before he walks out the door. Staying up late and reading a good book after the rest of my family is in deep slumber. Waking up to sleepy smiles, waffle sticks and SpongeBob SquarePants. Pushing Sophie in the stroller, while holding Jessica's hand as we cross the parking lot toward Baskin-Robbins. Collecting rocks along the beach, looking for the moon, hearing my daughter pray, watching my newborn baby smile in her sleep. Feeling my husband pull me close to him during the night. And, knowing what it means to be a mother, a wife, a *teacher*, a *writer* and a *dancer*.

Beverly Tribuiani-Montez

LIFE LESSON #3:
SANCTIFY THE ORDINARY

Many women go blithely about their days absorbed in their preoccupations until a crisis or some vague internal stirring stops them long enough to focus their attention on the deeper meaning in their lives.

How you do anything is how you do everything.

Zen saying

Shift your perspective—shift your

consciousness to see the sacred in the mundane. Regardless of your form of worship or belief, your spirituality shouldn't be something you devote yourself to only a few designated times each week. It should encompass your life, minute-by-minute, day-by-day.

Conscious/känshəs/ *awake and aware of one's surroundings and identity.*

Children are our greatest teachers. They mirror back to us our opportunities for growth (whether we want them to or not). If we choose, any relationship, any situation or any circumstance can also serve as our teacher.

You may think that learning is limited to the classroom, but why not consider your life a 24/7 seminar? Using life as your teacher is about paying attention to everything that occurs during your day. It's a matter of being mindful of your interactions, your reactions, and what they tell you about yourself and your life. The Buddha said to his disciples, "Be a light unto yourself."

Make the most routine tasks opportunities for contemplation. Whether you're picking up your children's clothes, washing dishes, talking with the postal clerk or vacuuming the floor, you can make everything you do sacred by investing it with care, consideration and compassion. As with anything else, you must commit yourself to this way of living daily. You can't do it once and forget about it. It requires effort and dedication.

We'd like to offer you a challenge. Why not see that God is in everything? In the food you cook for your family, the laundry you wash, the good-bye kisses you give your son or daughter as they go off to school. When you stop and think about it, doesn't it seem foolish to think that God is only present in a house of worship and not everywhere, in everything?

Everything you do matters—yes, everything. No act is too small or insignificant. You must live as if this is the truth. When you do, your life will become your spiritual practice.

Every interaction I have, every task I undertake,
everything that I do, matters.

The Dining Room Table

The deep brown mahogany of the dining room table was burnished with the soft patina of age and loving care. If wood could talk, it would tell the stories of Sunday dinners, birthday parties and hundreds of other family celebrations that spanned four generations. Krista remembered well the first time she had sat at this table at the home of her in-laws-to-be. The wonder of polishing it in her own home as a young bride. She pictured each of her children joining the family circle around it, in high chairs, youth chairs, and finally—"big chairs." How many birthdays, Christmases, Thanksgivings they had shared the bounty around it!

In just a few days, the table would be moving again, returning to her former husband for his new home and life. Of all the belongings that had been divided, this was the hardest to part with, she realized. To her, it represented a family gathered—traditions, continuity. Things that were not hers anymore. She couldn't imagine how her children would feel when the movers came. She had been able to rearrange the furniture in most of the other rooms, filling in gaps. But when the dining room table moved out, it would leave a huge hole—one she couldn't afford to fill. Yet how, she wondered, could she not provide the place of community and sharing that was also a part of what this table represented?

Suddenly she knew! "Meet me in the dining room," she called to Betsy, twelve, Ben, fourteen, and Karen, almost seventeen. When they were seated around the table, looking at her curiously, she said, "You know, this table belonged to your dad's grandparents and great-grandparents, so it is going to live with him. We have all had wonderful times around this table, and we're going to have a going-away party for it Saturday night. I want you each to invite two of your favorite friends over, and let's plan a menu we'll all enjoy . . ."

Saturday night came quickly. Soon they were twelve gathered around the antique banquet table, its leaves extended once more in welcome. Three middle-schoolers, six high-schoolers and three adults told stories of birthday parties and dinners and homework sessions, and the making of valentines and wrapping presents. They laughed. They remembered.

Just before dessert, Krista asked if everyone would join in clearing the table completely. When it was bare down to its exquisite surface, a dozen pair of hands carried the table to the garage. Then a dozen pair of hands lifted the "new" secondhand table Krista and the kids had discovered in a thrift shop, and carried it into the dining room. Carefully they laid it with the finest linen, silver and china, along with an array of decorations they had individually created just for this night. They lit candles, turned on the music and pulled their chairs around the table.

Krista lifted her glass and looked around the circle. "I want to propose a toast—to friends we love, who make our table a place of celebration! And to all of the celebrations to come!"

And so it was a grand celebration. An ending, a continuation—and a new beginning.

Kay Collier McLaughlin

LIFE LESSON #4: SEE THE POSITIVE

The true measure of a man is how he treats someone who can do him absolutely no good.

Samuel Johnson

How many times have you felt enraged at your ex-husband or boss? How many times have you felt frustrated with a friend or relative? Don't worry—we all have from time to time.

The next time you have these feelings, rather than

wishing they would disappear from your life, why not see your interactions as a catalyst? Ask yourself, Does this person challenge my authority by questioning my decisions? Do they demand more of me than I am willing to give? Why not use these relationships to grow stronger in your convictions and to practice standing up for yourself?

You have a choice about how you want to view every situation. You can see the irritation as an undeserved aggravation or as an opportunity. While these interactions may feel more like sandpapering than growth, you can choose to use them to polish your rough edges and strengthen yourself. The choice lies in your attitude. This means making a major shift in your thinking, but you'll find the results of this shift well worth the effort.

The philosopher Gurdjieff founded a spiritual community in France. Along with the students lived an old man whom no one liked. The man fought with everyone, refused to participate with the upkeep of the community, was rude and argumentative. After several months the man grew tired of how he was being treated and he packed up his belongings and left for Paris. All of the community members were greatly relieved. But not Gurdjieff.

He sought out the man and offered to pay him a sizeable monthly salary if he would come back to the community. When Gurdjieff returned with the man, everyone was horrified. When they learned that the old man was being paid for his bad manners while they were paying a stiff tuition to be part of the community, they became infuriated.

After hearing their complaints, Gurdjieff responded, "This man is like yeast for bread. Without him here you would never really learn about anger, irritability, patience and compassion. That is why you pay me, and that is why I hired him."

The people who annoy you the most and whom you find the most challenging to deal with are often your best teachers. The people whom you find the most irritating offer you an opportunity to become more introspective and aware. The next time you find yourself in a difficult situation— fuming at a coworker or ready to shriek at your spouse, partner or child—ask yourself, What does this person have to teach me?

We've all had experiences that we would have preferred to have avoided—conflicts at work, being caught at the airport with flight delays, illness, financial difficulties, to name but a few. These are what we call gifts in black wrapping paper—gifts that come whether we want them or not.

One of the magnificent things about human beings is that we have the ability to choose. Perhaps you can't change the external circumstances, but you can choose how you perceive a situation and how you approach it. The problem is not the problem, it's how you cope with a situation that makes it either positive or negative. Events in and of themselves can either be good or bad, but what's important is what you make of them. If you decide to live your life more consciously, then everything—yes, everything—becomes an opportunity for growth and transformation.

One of the characteristics of maturity is recognizing that the outcome of any given situation is far less important than how you cope with the challenge. The next time you find yourself in a tricky situation, challenge yourself to wring every ounce of meaning out of the circumstance—no matter how disappointing, how unpleasant, how discouraging—no matter what. Use everything in your life to learn more about yourself.

I am using everything in my life to learn more about myself and to create more of what I want.

Basic Tool: Daily Review

Before bed, sit quietly and go back over your day. Notice any areas of upset or disturbance and think about the understanding you can bring to the situation. Now consider five situations or circumstances in your life that you see as negative or as problems. Reframe them so that you think about the benefits you've reaped from dealing with each of these situations. Taking a few minutes at the end of each day gives you time to slow down and appreciate the lessons each day provides.

☕ A Turning Point

It is very easy to forgive others their mistakes;
it takes more grit and gumption to forgive
them for having witnessed your own.

JESSAMYN WEST

As everything unraveled on a twenty-five-year marriage and my husband moved out of the only home our daughter had ever known, I felt huge relief that our only child was twenty by that time—it made everything simpler. Or so I thought. Because she wasn't a minor, I didn't have to negotiate about custody and child support, didn't have to put up with his coming around to see her, didn't have to try to explain the inexplicable to a young child. Mostly, though, I was relieved because I thought it would be less complicated emotionally for her at that age. She was away at college, a young adult, not subject to the day-to-day difficulties or emotional turmoil of her parents being in two households.

In an attempt to ensure that my crushing hurt did not affect their relationship, I had said to my daughter and her dad that the nature and quality of their relationship from that point on would be up to them. I would not interfere, but neither would I facilitate. I tried to be glad when I saw his phone number on the phone bill from her college dorm; but I'll confess that on a few occasions in those early days I slipped into revenge fantasies, wishing with more than a little shame that I could be one of "those" divorced parents who use their children to "get at" an ex-spouse. My anger waned in intensity over the following months, but on occasion glowed white hot, briefly and unexpectedly, for reasons that still elude me. At those times, I exercised that remarkable ability so many women have to feign: pleasantness and serenity while simultaneously holding down an ugly knot of hurt and anger that clamored for attention the way curdled milk waits to erupt from a soured stomach.

I observed my daughter's next few years mostly from afar as she concentrated on her studies, became active in a sorority, made new friends, played on her university's tennis team, enjoyed snow-skiing, camping, boating and beach trips with friends, and fell in and out of love. I naturally wondered at times what impact the end of her parents' twenty-five-year marriage might have on her. From what I could see, my daughter's strong spirit, sense of independence, self-confidence, good humor and zest for life were serving her well. After a while, I even congratulated myself on our having handled things in a way that left her relatively unscathed.

Reality hit hard one evening during her Christmas vacation six months before she was to graduate from college. That's when my daughter taught me an important lesson—children whose parents divorce are forever changed, regardless of their age or life situation when the split happens. Sitting at the dinner table that night in my new house, which still didn't feel like home to either of us, she hesitantly told me she was dreading her college graduation.

"All my friends' families will be coming, and there are dinners and receptions all weekend," she said, putting her elbows on the table her father had sanded and stained when she was a little girl. "And every time you see Dad or talk about him, you cry and feel sad. I can't tell one of you not to come. You're my parents. It makes me not want to go through graduation."

I felt as though I'd been hit with something big and hard.

I couldn't breathe. And then tears—those damn tears—began to course down my cheeks and drip onto my chest. I felt hot, and the light over the table seemed to spin and flash as I struggled for composure. I was stunned and stung—stunned to discover that my involuntary tears had cut so deeply into her life and soul, stung that my hanging on to sadness and sense of loss were responsible for her wanting to skip an important milestone in her life. I didn't believe for a second she really would miss the festivities, but to know she saw my continued grieving as an inevitable dark cloud over her graduation weekend was devastating.

I've always believed that actions follow thoughts. Now would come a test of that belief. "I know it wasn't easy to say that," I managed to mutter. After a pause and a big sigh I continued, with a note of determination in my voice that I didn't feel. "It's six months until graduation. You know both your dad and I love you and want your graduation and all your special moments in life to be unmarred by what's gone on between us. I promise you that on your graduation week-end, you don't have to worry about my crying. We'll be fine."

And we were. Tears did fall that day, but they were shared with my ex-husband as we stood arm in arm watching the daughter we'd raised walk across the stage to accept her diploma. He even carried an extra handkerchief for me, as he had all those years we were married. That's when I knew my choice to spend time with him during the months after her sad dinner table confrontation had been worthwhile. By "practicing" being cordial and friendly, by sharing everyday conversation and meals, by saying why I was doing this, I had moved beyond the automatic response of tears. I think we actually ended up enjoying ourselves; and it wasn't long before I realized that forgiveness had crept into my heart, softening that hard knot of anger and hurt.

It was a turning point—not only for the three of us but for our extended family and friends as well. Now my sister and mother and friends could once again be friendly without feeling disloyal to me. The cordiality and friendliness we felt that spring has continued in the years since, making subsequent visits with our daughter more enjoyable for everyone. And now we're all immersed in planning another milestone—our daughter's wedding. In the fall, my ex-husband and I will sit side by side once again, on the front pew in the church this time, perhaps sharing a handkerchief once more.

A beloved teacher once said to me, "Forgiving may help the forgiver more than the forgiven." She was right.

Susan Carver Williams

LIFE LESSON #5:
LEARN TO FORGIVE

Living a life you love means extending love, compassion and forgiveness to the world. As you embrace your own imperfections, the ways in which you've disappointed and failed yourself, you discover greater understanding and self-acceptance. When you realize that you are just as capable of causing hurt, speaking out in anger and making mistakes as the next person, then you can begin to become more forgiving of yourself and others.

You've been angry at your parents, siblings, spouses, children or friends. But let's face it, you're not going to make them redo the past. You have a choice. You can either hold on to your anger and allow it to poison your life, or you can find a way to let go of your old grudges.

It's no small feat to forgive those who have hurt you. But when you put yourself in their shoes and understand the desperation, fear or ignorance that was the origin of their actions—when you truthfully consider whether you could have done or have done something similar—it becomes easier to forgive.

When you refuse to forgive, you're pretending that you aren't as flawed as the rest of humanity. Forgiveness insists that you admit you're just like every other human being doing the best they can with what they presently know. Forgiveness requires you to open your heart to the suffering of others.

No snowflake in an avalanche ever feels responsible.

Voltaire

I am forgiving those who have hurt me and experiencing greater freedom and healing.

☕ Counting Laps

Gratitude unlocks the fullness of life.
It turns what we have into enough, and more . . .
It can turn a meal into a feast, a house into
a home, a stranger into a friend.

MELODY BEATTIE

In 2002 my dad, brother, sister and I bought a small condo in Florida. Being faint-of-pocketbook, my quarter-share took most of my retirement money, but I live by the principle that you should follow your dreams while you're still awake. Besides, I was born in Tallahassee just two months after the big war ended and I've always thought God intended for me to be a Floridian, even though my folks moved back to their home state of Illinois three weeks after my birth and I've lived up north ever since.

At any rate, I'm happier than a flower-lover in a field full of orchids every time I get to stay at the family condo. Florida has captured my heart. No matter how many times I make the trip, I am thrilled to arrive in sun, sand, sea, surf and swimming pool country.

The large condo pool is next to the Intracoastal Waterway, one street away from the Gulf of Mexico. Every day I swim. Sometimes I swim two or three times a day. And each time I'm at the pool, I'm actually in the water, unlike most people who sit in the lounge chairs reading, talking or sleeping. Not me. I go to the pool to swim, and I'm often in the water for an hour-and-a-half or two hours at a time, swimming leisurely laps. My goal is thirty lengths or fifteen laps per session. Sometimes I double that.

The problem with swimming laps is keeping track. My mind wanders. *Oh, look, there's a dolphin jumping out of the Intracoastal!* Or three or four condo friends jump in the pool to cool off and we gab each time I reach the shallow end. Or perhaps a pelican, seagull, heron or egret swoops by to my delight when I'm doing the backstroke and I lose track of my lap count.

My cousin Meta has one solution for keeping track of laps. She walks around her one-eighth mile circular drive-way out in the country every morning twenty-four times with her neighbor. Meta has a large coffee can on the driveway that holds twenty-four small pebbles. When they start walking she puts the pebbles in her coat pocket and drops one in the can each time they go around. As these two women chat about everything under their Cincinnati sky, they know exactly when they've finished their three miles.

But at the swimming pool, there's no place in my swimsuit for thirty pebbles. The solution came one day when I was feeling especially joyful about being in that pool under a robin's egg blue sky on a glorious 80-degree Florida day. I started thanking God for all my blessings. *That's it!* I thought. *I'll think about specific blessings that have particular importance in my life and that have significance to the number of lap I'm on.*

ONE: One God gave me life, and it's up to me to use this one life to the fullest. Side stroke, breaststroke, crawl. I praise God for granting me so many blessings. Me, a single parent who marches through life as one woman, not as a couple. Thank you, Lord, for giving me life.

TWO: On this lap I think about how fortunate I am to have two homes and that my brother, sister, their families, my folks and I are so close that we can make a joint-owner vacation condo work so happily for all of us. Two homes, one up north, one down south. It doesn't get any better than that, Lord.

THREE: Lap number three is about the work I do. Again the Lord has blessed me with work I love. Three part-time freelance jobs, instead of one monumental stressful one. I write, I speak, I paint jars. I make a little money with each job, enough to survive. Lots of freedom. Breaststroke, frog kick. Thank you, Lord, for giving me the ability to do this work and to love my three jobs so much.

FOUR: My four children—two daughters, two sons. Children who have filled my life with joy, sometimes angst. But, oh, the blessings of having children. As I butterfly kick my way to the other end of the pool, I think about each child. Jeanne's recent marriage and move to California. Julia's struggles as a single parent. Michael's busy life with the university band and his growing family. Andrew's determination to finish college while working his dream job for ESPN Sports. Four interesting lives. Suddenly that lap is finished.

FIVE: I wonder what I'm thankful for that has a number five connected to it. Sometimes it's hard to come up with something for a certain number. One day in the pool I recalled that I have five pairs of sandals in my condo closet. Wow, Lord, thank you for the variety of footwear you have blessed me with. The next day as I did the side stroke up the pool and down, I praised the Lord for a tasty five-bean salad I made and for the five friends who ate it.

SIX: Six grandchildren. Three blondes, three redheads. Hailey, Casey, Riley, Hannah, Zachary and Chloe. I love lap number six best. Imagine the fun of thinking about the antics of six little people who are tied so tightly to your heartstrings that sometimes you think you'll just burst from happiness.

SEVEN: The seven seas. As a swimmer I pass the time back-stroking during lap seven by recalling all the wonderful places I've swum—Atlantic, Pacific, the aquamarine Caribbean, the Gulf of Mexico, the warm waters off Kauai, Oahu and the big island of Hawaii. Lord, thank you for the seven seas, the oceans, rivers, lakes and ponds. Thank you for water.

EIGHT: One time when I was on lap number eight, I started thinking about figure eights in ice-skating. I hadn't ice-skated for years and never could do a figure eight, but I still count my blessings for all the fun winter sports I enjoyed in my youth up north.

NINE: The first thing that came to mind when I hit lap number nine was "nine lives" as in the number cats are supposed to have. Often when I'm in Florida, my friends Wally and Shirley are on vacation somewhere else so I get to take care of their cats, Bubba and Boomer. The "boys," as I call them, and I get along famously, and I'm always happy if I get cat duty so they can keep me company. Lord, please give Bubba and Boomer at least nine lives.

TEN: This is the place in my lap swimming where I examine my conscience. The ten commandments come in handy for this one. I run through them all, trying to decide if I've blown it and whether or not I need to apologize to anyone for anything.

Sometimes I only do ten laps. Sometimes twenty. Now that I've figured out how to keep track of the count, my pool time takes on a life of its own. Every day I get out of that pool a new person . . . blessings counted, prayers said, conscience examined, life evaluated, attitude adjusted and exercise completed.

Jump in! The water's perfect!

Patricia Lorenz

LIFE LESSON #6: ACKNOWLEDGE YOUR BLESSINGS

There is an ancient custom in Thailand for expressing gratitude. On the grounds of the temples throughout the country are hundreds of brass bowls. Each person who walks past the offering bowl drops a coin into it. As the coin rings, they say something for which they are grateful.

An American woman was visiting one of these temples and as she walked around the temple grounds she followed this custom. As she paused at the first bowl she said, "I'm grateful for my family." At the second bowl she said, "I'm thankful for my health." In bowls three, four and five she expressed gratitude for her love of music, the natural world, her spiritual life. Then she panicked.

The woman saw countless bowls before her and she was afraid that she had run out of things for which to be grateful. She stood for a moment searching her mind for yet another blessing. After a few minutes the woman was flooded with how much she had in her life for which to give thanks. With this new realization the woman approached the next bowl, and the next, and completed the process.

It is inevitable when one has a great need of something, one finds it. What you need you attract to you like a lover.

Gertrude Stein

The woman decided that before she returned home she would purchase a brass bowl. To this day she continues this ritual. Every morning she acknowledges the small kindnesses, the little noticed blessings of everyday life. As a result of this experience, she discovered that the blessings are everywhere she chooses to look. She simply had to learn to recognize them.

All too often you focus on what you don't have, what you can't afford, what's missing from your life. You want more, when you don't genuinely appreciate what you already have. When you shift your perspective you realize how much you have to be grateful for.

As you recognize the richness of your life, stop for a moment and give thanks. Give thanks for life itself. Give thanks for all of your resources—your ability to see, to hear, to taste, to touch, to speak. Your ability to think, to feel, to love, to laugh. There is so much for which to be thankful. Focus each and every day on what you have—on what's right with your life—and express your gratitude. Your life will be enriched immensely by this simple practice.

I am continually aware of all of the blessings in my life.

Questions Worth Asking

- Are my basic needs taken care of?
- Do I have shelter, food and clothing?
- Do I have family and friends I can count on?
- Can I go to the movies, watch a sunset, listen to my favorite piece of music, eat delicious food, smell the fragrance of fresh cut flowers, feel the warmth of the sun on my face?

⫯⫯ The Finishing Touch

GRATITUDE INVENTORY

Make a list of all the things you're grateful for. Consider the various areas of your life. Think about your family, your friends, your home, your work, your appearance, your education, your talents, your health—the possibilities are endless.

Consider how each situation, relationship or circumstance enriches your life. And as you do, allow yourself to take in what each of these blessings means to you.

For the next week, make a commitment to start each day by giving thanks for at least three things for which you are grateful. You may also want to pause throughout the day when you recognize another blessing and silently give thanks. At the end of the week, notice how you feel. This sense of gratitude will shift your focus from what you think is missing in your life to a greater appreciation for all that you have.

Essential Ingredient

SHARE THE LOVE

We cannot do great things on this Earth.
We can only do small things
with great love.

Mother Teresa

We Celebrated a Life

It was the final three weeks, as I look back, of the life of my husband and companion of nearly fifty-eight years. It had been only three weeks since he had been diagnosed with a fast-acting lung cancer which had already spread to lymph glands. He was rapidly growing weaker, but we were determined that he would die at home as he wished.

With the help of hospice, on call as we needed medicines, equipment or instructions, I was managing. But there seemed no way to keep cheer in and despair out of my attitude. We discussed his dying. After all, he was eighty-six years old. We were reconciled to the facts. Our years together had been very satisfying with more positive events than negative. Our three children and grandchildren were blessings and sources of great pride. We had shared many celebrations and happy times, and had survived the sorrow of losing our son Michel who had been killed in a car wreck when he was forty-six. He left a wife and two sons who, eventually, added to our contentment.

So, living day by day, knowing one would soon be his last, we walked one last unknown path together. As I watched the consciousness of his world grow smaller, I found myself wondering about life and its purposes.

I had taught school for forty years, grades one through university, before retiring. Had I really made a difference? Did I make a permanent, positive effect on any one of those lives that came through my classrooms? Had the friendly, jolly man who was my husband brought encouragement and hope to anyone?

Our daughter Melissa had come to be with us for a few days. Husband Ray had been able to sit at the table and eat breakfast that morning. We had just gotten him to his recliner when the doorbell announced a florist delivery. It was a big beautiful bouquet of pink roses with a card that read:

"Mr. and Mrs. Clendenin, if I had a flower for all the times you have made me laugh or smile, I would have a flower garden to walk through for the rest of my life. Just wanted you to know how much I love and appreciate you two."

The card was unsigned.

Trying to guess who sent the tribute, I was determined to be kind to all our acquaintances!

Melissa and I decided to go by the florist shop and see if the omission of the name had been intentional or accidental. The lady at the shop checked out the receipt.

No name. And the order was by wire, not local. She promised to do some tracing to determine if the sender wanted
to remain unknown.

Next morning I had an e-mail from the superintendent of
a small school in New Mexico. He said, "You two are the
most wonderful people that God blessed us with when we
first came to the United States."

Turns out, when that family with eight children moved to
our little town of Cloudcroft, New Mexico, Miguel and his
sister were placed in the class with our Melissa. Neither of
the new students spoke English, but they learned quickly.
Melissa and Rosa were soon best friends all through grade
school, high school and college, and even now. The entire
family became close friends with our family.

Miguel, the oldest child, was the only one born in Mexico.
I helped him get his citizenship and grants for college when
he was graduated from high school. Then, all eight children
earned degrees. Besides the superintendent, one is a bank
vice-president, one a director of special education for three
counties, one a bank auditor (before retiring to stay home
with her children), one a buyer for a research corporation,
and the others are well established also.

Miguel's was the first of several letters we got from the
family.

Others began to remember us, too. One former student
said, "I should have told you how much I appreciated you

a long time ago. You helped me as a student and as a colleague. I am who I am because of you and others who helped me gain confidence."

Another, a high school principal in Arizona, wrote to share good news of her success as a first-year principal in a school that had been an underachieving school when she was assigned there. The school was practically run by gangs before she assumed control, winning over students and teachers, and convincing them that education improved life and that she really cared. At the end of the year, when test scores came in showing significant gain, enough to remove them from underachieving to positive status, she celebrated with more than 2,300 students and teachers. The last paragraph of her letter was:

"It made me think back to my university days, when my English teacher there did not think I was good enough to be a teacher. Yet, you did, and advocated for me. You saw something in me that I did not even see in myself. You believed in me when I did not, and you loved me when I needed it the most. You truly turned my life around. They say the impact of a great teacher sometimes is not realized until many years down the road. I guess I am living proof of this. Here I am years later thanking my teacher for the impact she had on my life. I love you! Thank you for saving my life."

That young lady came to Lubbock Christian University, Lubbock, Texas, from New York knowing no one here. Becoming a family friend, she asked Ray to give her away when she was married. We were Papa C and Mama C to her.

There were others. So many expressions of appreciation for Ray's friendly smile and handshake which made them feel favored. Always some humor to share, he was a friend to everyone.

One young man who had come to church reluctantly with his parents and is now a grown man said, "Mr. Clendenin was my friend. He made me feel as if he really cared."

So, on November 24, we truly celebrated a life lived, not ended. More than 200 people came to celebrate and to assure me that our lives did have meaning. We sang songs that he had loved and sung. The hallelujahs rang! He did make a difference. We did touch a few lives. We celebrated!

The tears still come unexpectedly sometimes, especially when yet another person assures me that our lives, our marriage, was a model for them. I tell my little dog and pretty black cat about plans for the day as we go for our morning walk. They seem to understand that we are blessed.

Mary Joe Clendenin

LIFE LESSON #1:
REMEMBER WHAT YOU HAVE TO OFFER

One of the primary messages of this book is to learn to put yourself first. You have to take care of your needs before you can take care of the needs of others. However, once you have a sense that your life is on track and your needs are being met, it's time to turn your attention to making a contribution to the larger community.

One must think like a hero to behave like a merely decent human being.

May Sarton

After all, caring is intrinsic to being human. It's a reflex. You live, therefore you care. A woman drops her package, you help her to gather her belongings; a blind person stands in a crosswalk, you offer to guide him across the street; a coworker is locked out of her car, you offer to call a locksmith. It's a natural part of being human. You live, therefore you help.

When disaster strikes or any emergency occurs, you are quick to lend a hand. We rally together during a flood, earthquake or fire. We bring food to a friend when a loved one passes away. We baby-sit for a neighbor when her parent is rushed to the hospital. Yet we don't have to wait for times of crisis to share our compassion. We can—in fact we must—share our caring on a regular basis.

You give to others for obvious moral reasons, but when you stop and think about it, service also enriches your life—you receive a gift in the giving. Have you ever noticed how you can be in a bad mood, but when someone calls you and you extend yourself, your mood shifts immediately? At those times, you're reminded of who you really are and what you have to offer. It's not just the person on the receiving end that benefits; you do as well.

Work and live to serve others, to leave the world a little better than you found it and garner for yourself as much peace of mind as you can. This is happiness.

David Sarnoff

Giving adds a sense of satisfaction to life that few other experiences can. When you reach out to others, you feel your interconnectedness with all of life. You feel a kinship, a sense of community—a taste of unity and belonging.

But you can't simply give once and expect that it will have a lasting effect. You have to make service a habit—a natural part of your everyday life. When you begin to give of yourself, you'll find that the old saying, "Virtue is its own reward," really does ring true.

I am recognizing my gifts and talents and using them to make a contribution.

☕ May Baskets

I looked always outside myself to see
what I could make the world give me instead of
looking within myself to see what was there.

BELLE LIVINGSTONE

It is May Day and the warm sunshine has finally coaxed my gardens into bloom. As my children carefully tuck tiny spring flowers into the bright paper baskets they will take to our neighbors, they beg me to tell them again the story of the years my sisters and I took May baskets to the witch.

Mrs. Pearson wasn't really a witch but she lived on our lane in an old gray cottage whose overgrown yard was enclosed by a sagging fence. Her gardens, Mother told us, were once the envy of the neighborhood. Now, we rarely saw her. At Halloween, she would place a bowl of candy on her porch and hide behind her faded curtains. When carolers came to her door at Christmas, her house remained silent and dark. But every year, when my little sisters and I made May baskets, Mother would urge us to take one to Mrs. Pearson.

Our other neighbors always made a great fuss. "Look, Arthur," Mrs. Peabody would call to her husband, "see what the fairies have left for us." Miss Addie Wilson, at the house across the road, must have listened for our quick knock for sometimes she almost caught us as we ran to hide behind her azalea. But Mrs. Pearson never opened her door. Year after year, our little baskets hung on her doorknob until the lilies dangled limply and the daisies turned brown.

The year I turned ten, I begged Mother to let us pass by Mrs. Pearson's house. She just quietly shook her head. "You may not think so, but I know your baskets bring joy to that lonely old lady." So, once again, Ellen and I, holding firmly to Beth's chubby little hand, crept up to her door, knocked rather half-heartedly, and scurried behind a bush. "This is silly," I whispered to Ellen. "She never comes out."

"Ssshhh," Ellen whispered fiercely, pointing toward the door as it slowly opened. A tiny white-haired lady stepped onto the porch. She removed the May basket from her doorknob and sat down on the top step, our basket in her lap. Suddenly, she put her face in her hands.

"Oh dear, she's crying!" said Beth, darting out. Mother had put Beth in our charge so Ellen and I quickly climbed up the steps after her. We found her gently patting Mrs. Pearson's shoulder.

"Are you all right?" I asked with concern.

"Yes, dear, I'm fine," she said as she looked up, wiping her cheek. "You don't know how much I love your little May baskets. I always leave them on the door so all the passersby can admire them." She paused and smiled shyly. "I just got a bit overwhelmed at the happy memories. You see, long ago, my sister and I used to make May baskets just like these."

Beth continued her patting.

"Would you girls like to come in and have some milk and graham crackers? I could show you pictures of when we were just about your age."

"Yes," declared Beth, marching through the open door. Since Mother had told us not to let her out of our sight, we followed.

As we sat in Mrs. Pearson's tidy little parlor eating our graham crackers, she showed us old photographs of her and her sister rolling hoops down sunlit hillsides, playing with their dolls in the woods, and best of all, the two of them, proudly holding their little paper May baskets trimmed with long ribbons.

I wish I could say that after our visit Mrs. Pearson began tending her garden again or that she answered the door at Halloween and admired our costumes, but she didn't. Nevertheless, for the next several years, until we grew too old to weave paper baskets and hide behind lilac bushes, each May Day, we would climb the steps to her porch and find a little basket just for us. It was full of cookies cut in the shape of flowers, with pink frosting and sugar sprinkles.

Faith Andrews Bedford

LIFE LESSON #2:
RECOGNIZE WHAT
YOU HAVE TO CONTRIBUTE

Many women feel that what they have to give wouldn't be enough to make a significant contribution. No matter what your background or training, no matter what your assessment of your gifts, talents or abilities, there is one thing that you undoubtedly possess—the most invaluable commodity —love. With that as your foundation we know that there is much more that you have to give. If you're uncertain, why not ask your family and friends what they think your gifts are? These attributes may be

Questions
Worth Asking

- If I could change one thing about the world, what would it be?

- If I won the lottery, with what organizations would I share the wealth?

- If I volunteered one day a month, where would it be? Why haven't I done this yet?

difficult for you to identify, but they're usually obvious to others.

It's time to take yourself in hand and find a way to contribute. Refer back to the list of positive qualities you identified in the first chapter and consider how you can use some of those talents and gifts to benefit others. Consider again your interests. What do you really value in life? What truly warms your heart? What can you do to turn these values and interests into action?

Giving can take many forms. You can start by cooking dinner for a sick friend, writing a letter to the editor, signing up for a food drive at your church, coaching a girls' soccer team, or helping to organize a voter registration drive. Giving is as easy as offering words of encouragement to the people you interact with on a daily basis, making thoughtful gestures, or extending common courtesies.

Basic Tool: Your Favorite Causes

Take out a sheet of paper and create two columns. In the first one, list your skills. Are you a good typist? Do you sew or cook well? Maybe you're a great public speaker or a wonderful writer. Do you have professional skills, like legal or medical knowledge? List at least five things you do well.

In the second columns, write down the issues or causes about which you truly care. Are you passionate about the rights of children? The environment? Teen pregnancy? Low-income housing? World hunger? Drunk driving? Freedom of speech? Your religion or spiritual beliefs? Again, list at least three issues that are near and dear to your heart.

What you've created is your giving preferences—your favorite causes. You have five skills that any organization would love for you to share with them. You have three issues for which you would love to share your talents and skills. Now go out there and find a way to make a contribution.

I am using my whole self
to be of service in the world.

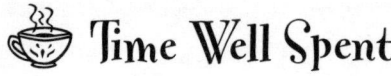 Time Well Spent

Keep a good heart.
That's the most important thing in life.
It's not how much money you make
or what you can acquire.
The art of it is to keep a good heart.

JONI MITCHELL

It was incredibly cold outside. The wind hurled through the southern tip of Manhattan right through the site of the World Trade Center towers. The once luminous buildings were no longer there to protect us from the bite of the bitter wind. And I, a Floridian—well, it seemed unbearable to me. Inside my head, I repeated over and over again, *I am so miserable. I am so miserable. I am so miserable.*

We were clothed in heavy coats, hard hats, orange safety vests and lots of identification or "credentials," as they say. We were on a mission trip to Ground Zero—to serve and assist those working during the clean-up efforts after the attacks on September 11, 2001. I looked to my right and saw some rescue workers raking in painstaking slow motion, looking for . . . well, you know. And then reality hit: *I don't even know the meaning of miserable, but those workers certainly do.*

I continued making my way around the sixteen-acre property, with my new friend, Mac, a volunteer chaplain for the NYPD. We offered water and hot chocolate to the rescue workers in and around "the pit." I didn't realize what a valuable commodity hot chocolate and water could be. Most of us in America can get a drink of water or hot chocolate any time of day. But these workers, in these conditions, could not just walk down the hall and get a much-needed drink during their grueling shifts on duty.

We came upon a trailer labeled "morgue." Oh my goodness—just the word made me want to run the other way. But something made me stop and knock on the door. The wind was blowing so hard, it hurt. The dust and rubble churning through the air made it hard to breathe. The door flew open. I was afraid to see what was inside this building so I kept my eyes fixed on the woman answering the door and asked, "Would you like some hot chocolate?"

"Hot chocolate! You're kidding," she stated. "I'd love some hot chocolate."

"With marshmallows?" I asked.

"You even have marshmallows?" She couldn't believe it. Her face lit up. Her name was Maryanne.

Later, I saw Maryanne taking a break in the basement of St. Peter's Church—a refuge for rescue workers and our home for a week. We chatted a bit. The following night I ran into her again at dinnertime. I was struck by the fact that this sweet lady with a gentle disposition worked in a morgue. Not any old morgue, but one right in the footprints of one of our country's most devastating war zones. I didn't want to think about what she'd seen over the last few months.

At the end of the week, I reported for my last official night shift working at Ground Zero. As I entered the basement of St. Peter's Church, I noticed Maryanne sitting at a table. Her face lit up when she saw me bounding down the steps. She said, "I've been looking for you." So I approached the table. "I've been looking for you," she repeated.

"Me? You've been looking for me?" I didn't really know her that well. I wasn't in charge of anything. Just serving. *What could she possibly want from me?*

"You've been looking for me?" I asked again.

"Oh yeah," she shrugged her shoulders, "I was just looking for ya."

Silence. I realized at that moment that Maryanne didn't have anything to say to me. No questions. No comments. Nothing. She was "just looking for me." She just wanted to see a friendly face. A smile.

Maryanne taught me an important life lesson that week at

Ground Zero. Often the greatest gift we can give someone is our time. Our presence can be quite a present, a very precious gift indeed.

I haven't seen Maryanne since that week. I wonder how she's doing. I wish I could spend some time with her again. Working on the night shift at Ground Zero was the worst experience of my life—but the lessons I learned in that pit will be treasures I'll carry with me forever. It certainly was time well spent.

Karen Fortner Granger

LIFE LESSON #3:
CULTIVATE COMPASSION

Compassion is the understanding that we're all interconnected. Despite our differences in race, socio-economic status, ethnicity or age, we are all essentially the same. We share the same dreams, fears, struggles, needs, hopes and joys. We share the common desire to attain fulfillment and avoid pain. When we strip away our outer façades, we are at heart one.

How lovely to think that no one need wait a moment, we can start now, start slowly changing the world!

Anne Frank

Many persons have a wrong idea of what constitutes real happiness. It is not obtained through self-gratification but through fidelity to a worthy purpose.

Helen Keller

The obstacles that separate us fall away when we realize we are the homeless person begging for food. We are the welfare mother worried about caring for her family. We are the alcoholic struggling for sobriety. We are the battered woman in need of a safe harbor.

Compassion helps you to recognize that everybody is doing the best they can with the information and tools they currently have. Compassion alleviates blame and allows you to accept other people as they are despite their differences.

The root of compassion begins at home, with yourself. If you are critical and hard on yourself, you tend to be critical of others. If you're compassionate and accepting of yourself, you tend to be more accepting of others.

Compassion\ kəm-'pash-ən
sympathetic consciousness of others' distress together with a desire to alleviate it.

How many of you walk around judging and criticizing other people? The truth is, we all do. It's our way of not having to admit that we are just as imperfect and fallible as the woman who screams at her child in the toy store, or the man who berates the waitress for bringing him the wrong order, or the woman who remains in an abusive marriage. We're all guilty of being critical. But pretending that we're better than other people only serves to keep us separate.

The expression of compassion can take many forms: You can donate your time, make a financial contribution or share your ideas. Compassion connects you with the larger community. It allows you to experience an intimate connection with another person, to be able to genuinely know their pain. It makes the world a smaller, less lonely place.

No matter what the situation, compassion is the appropriate response. Can you stretch yourself to be more than you ever thought you could be? Can you find within a greater generosity than you thought you were capable of? And as challenging as this may sound, compassion isn't enough. You must take action. You must put your caring and concern into practice.

*I am compassionate with myself,
my loved ones and everyone with whom
I come in contact.*

Basic Tool: Places to Get Involved

When you feel compelled to extend your gifts and take action, a good place to start is *www.volunteermatch.com*. There are organizations throughout the country that could be great outlets to express your compassion. Browse the site and find an organization that interests you. If you're not ready to volunteer your time just yet, take a minute to simply take a peek at the myriad ways to get involved. When you are ready, you'll have some ideas for ways to get started. If you do not have access to the Internet, look in your local newspaper or ask your local librarian for volunteer opportunities in your community.

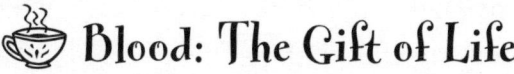 Blood: The Gift of Life

We cannot hold a torch to light another person's
path without brightening our own.

BEN SWEETLAND

I was still chuckling as I left the Red Cross blood drive today with my two younger children in tow. As I'd gathered our coats, someone had turned to me and said, "I hear you have four young children. Why do you give blood?"

"Are you kidding?" I laughed. "When I donate, the volunteers watch my children, they feed me, they tell me how wonderful I am and I get to put my feet up for twenty minutes. It's a great deal."

Left unsaid was my other reason for giving; the reason that still chills me when I allow myself to remember. It was eighteen months ago at what was supposed to be the routine delivery of another healthy Cram baby. But this baby was different. Just moments before birth, something went terribly wrong: I suffered a rare amniotic embolism, which collapsed my blood's clotting system.

As the baby made her rapid appearance into the world,

medical personnel scurried around with worried looks and hushed voices. My husband stood by helplessly as he heard, "Not much time . . . extremely critical . . . prep more blood . . . can't promise we can save her . . ." Grueling hours later, after emergency surgery and transfusions, he heard the sweet news that I was one of the lucky ones, one of the 14 percent who survive this complication. It had taken the speed and skill of eight doctors, and the availability of twenty-five units of blood.

A year and a day later I became eligible to donate blood again, and I could scarcely contain my excitement. My husband was baffled. How could I explain it to him? Somewhere out there are twenty-five people who bared their arms, flinched for a brief moment, then watched (or didn't watch) as a pint of their life's blood was freely offered. All they received in return were some kind words and a cup of juice from Red Cross volunteers.

Those twenty-five people did not donate because it was convenient. They had to leave work early or juggle a car pool schedule or miss dinner that night. It's not that they had nothing better to do. They donated blood because they knew that their pint of blood could make a difference, and maybe even save a life.

Mine is the life they saved. You'd never know it if you saw me. I am just another overwhelmed mother who looks healthy and exhausted, but those twenty-five people helped to ensure that a baby will grow up hearing the sound of her mother's laughter, that a young father could bring his wife home to grow old with him. Somewhere out there today, in some hospital corridor, is another terrified young husband, or parent, or sister, or friend, desperately hoping that his loved one survives, and that loved one looks an awful lot like me.

So I gave blood today, and my toddler and preschooler came to watch to see if Mama's blood is red, just like last time, or if this time it's green. They got bandages on their arms to match mine, and stickers, and a glimpse of the gift of life. We ate cookies and drank our milk, and I left with a little less blood and a much fuller heart. You see, I gave blood today, and all I felt was good.

M. Regina Cram

LIFE LESSON #4:
THE BLESSING OF GIVING

Giving is its own reward. Service to others is an act of reverence and gratitude for the life you are living. As you recognize the richness of everyday life, there is a natural impulse to want to give back to the world. It's an outgrowth of leading a rich and fulfilling life. Get into the habit of making a contribution to the greater community. Cultivate your innate caring and compassion. Share the wealth of all that you are and all that you have.

Our impact far exceeds what each of us can contribute individually. Making a contribution no matter how small sets off a chain reaction. Each person you affect passes on the kindness and caring to another person. As a result, your actions have a domino effect.

Your contributions can take many forms from grand, far-reaching actions to simple acts of kindness. As you take steps towards creating a life you love, you will find yourself giving more and more. You will give by what you do. You will give by striving for your dreams. You will give by sharing your experiences and knowledge. In effect, your life becomes a message of compassion, encouragement and inspiration.

Gratitude unlocks the fullness of life. It turns what we have into enough, and more. It turns denial into acceptance, chaos into order, confusion to clarity. It can turn a meal into a feast, a house into a home, a stranger into a friend. Gratitude makes sense of our past, brings peace for today, and creates vision for tomorrow.

Melody Beattie

The question now is, How can you use the wisdom you've gained from your life to better the planet? How can you give back to the world a portion of its lost heart? While most of us have come to realize that we aren't going to change the world, what we can—in fact, what we *must* do—is something, anything, to make a difference . . . one small step at a time.

As I reach out to others, I experience the gifts that service brings.

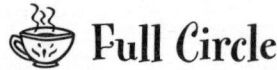 Full Circle

I own my life. And only mine.
And so I shall appreciate my person.
And so I shall make proper use of myself.

RUTH BEEBE HILL

A nearly full moon hangs low on the horizon, buttery yellow and hung with the shred of cobweb clouds. My footsteps stir the tang of fallen leaves. Woodsy, smoke-scented shouts of distant children drift on newly chill air. I lift the lid on a carved pumpkin and inexpertly light the candle inside. This watershed event is witnessed only by a passing ghoul who is clueless to the fact that this is the first year I've been deemed grown-up enough to do this job totally on my own. But the significance isn't lost on me. I importantly monitor the flickering flame inside the jack-o-lantern and feel suddenly grown-up. I'm ten years old and responsible enough to use matches unsupervised to light a pumpkin I carved by myself with a real knife. In a few minutes I'll even be going trick-or-treating with friends and not parents for the first time in my life.

Euphoria fizzes through my body. I lose some of my elation by racing, skipping and dancing around our front yard, safe in its familiarity but exhilarated by its transformation to shadow, mist and moonlight. I am giddy on the rite-of-passage incense of scorched pumpkin.

Twenty-five years later, a nearly full moon hangs low on the horizon on a Halloween evening. I'm in a different house now, in a different state. Being "big" isn't quite as exciting as it once was. But the smells are the same. Earth, dew, leaf, smoke, flame. The scents of nostalgia. As usual, I am the self-appointed lighter-of-pumpkins. And this year my own children are old enough to be interested in my ritual. They crowd around: two medieval princesses and a knight in shining armor, jockeying for a good view. "Can I do the next one?" one of them asks eagerly. A chorus of, "Me, me, I want to do it!" ensues. I inform them they aren't big enough yet. "Well, when will we be big enough?" one of my three-year-olds want to know.

"Maybe when you're ten," I say, remembering. "That's forever!" Rapunzel wails. I know otherwise, but I don't argue. Instead, I divert the conversation. "Hey guys! Who's ready to go trick-or-treating?!" As one, the three of them jump up and down shouting, "I am! I am!" If they were any more enthusiastic, they'd wriggle right out of their skins and shoot up into the sky like tiny bottle rockets. Instead they start racing around the yard after each other, not straying far from the safe pools of shadowy light cast by the lamppost and the jack-o-lanterns. In the thrall of their excitement, I feel suddenly un-grown-up, suddenly ten again. There is that same surge of euphoria, and I lose some of my elation by joining my children in their mad dance around the front yard.

Pretty soon we're shrieking, laughing, howling, cavorting in the mist and the moonlight. "Mommy! Look how big we are! We're not even scared of the dark!" one of them shouts exultantly. How big indeed.

And they, newly big, and I, newly little, dance on in the shadows of our common ground, intoxicated on the smell of scorched pumpkins.

Karen C. Driscoll

LIFE LESSON #5:
CELEBRATE, CELEBRATE

As you come to the end of this book, you are to be congratulated on the steps you've taken to create a more fulfilling life. Very few women are comfortable acknowledging their accomplishments. They simply gloss over them and move on to the next challenge. They rarely slow down long enough to notice that they've changed. They fail to appreciate that through small incremental steps, they've actually made significant changes in their lives.

You may feel shy about calling too much attention to yourself. The idea of celebrating the changes you've made both internally and externally may feel awkward. However, it's important to acknowledge what you've accomplished and how much you've grown. Encouragement and acknowledgment nurture the seeds for future change.

Many people underestimate the effort involved in creating a quality life. Do something that signals your acceptance and appreciation for where you are in your life and how far you've come. Buy yourself a bouquet of flowers, write yourself a letter of appreciation or take yourself out to lunch.

There are certain characteristics of women who choose to live an authentic life. Here are some of the qualities these remarkable women exhibit.

Authentic women are:

Willing to own what they know, what they've experienced and who they are.

Connected to their passion, vitality, wisdom and individuality.

Free to express their thoughts, feelings and needs.

Connected to their inner strength.

Living their lives with integrity, and assuming responsibility for themselves, their fulfillment and their actions.

Honoring their bodies as the temples of their spirits.

The primary subjects of their own lives.

Pursuing their dreams.

Exhibiting a capacity for love, understanding and compassion.

Aware of their interconnectedness with life and compelled to make a meaningful contribution to the world, not from a place of obligation, but from a place of fullness.

And finally, an authentic woman trusts herself.

This is the woman you are becoming.

The world is a better place because you are one of its cherished citizens. No question about it. Give yourself a message of appreciation for the caring, committed, loving woman you truly are. Start with this simple message: "I love me, I value me." Say it to yourself every day or whenever you need a little boost. People are starved for recognition. You're no different. You will blossom under this kind of acknowledgment. It may feel awkward at first. Most women have been

Gratitude is the heart's memory.

French Proverb

trained to tell other people that they are loved and valued. Some might consider it selfish to lavish this kind of attention on themselves. But it's long overdue.

Consider how different your day would be if you woke up and said a loving phrase to yourself first thing each morning. Think of this as a one-a-day vitamin for your soul. Be proud of who you truly are. Embrace yourself in your entirety—the woman who encompasses all that you do and all that you are.

Make a commitment to start each day with this personal message of appreciation. Give thanks for all your blessings. And start now to live the life you were meant to live.

I am celebrating the ways in which I have grown and the woman I am becoming.

The Finishing Touch

THE LIFE YOU LOVE

Make a list of all the ways you've changed during the course of reading this book. Do you make more time for yourself now? Have you made yourself more of a priority? Are you more confident? Do you say "no" and set limits more easily? Have you discovered your passion and made it a part of your everyday life? Do you live more simply? Are you more willing to ask for support, advice and assistance? Do you nurture your connections with friends and family? Have you discovered ways to make every day sacred?

Make a list of ten ways in which you have improved your life. They can range from small, barely perceptible changes to more significant accomplishments. *Progress, not perfection, is what's important.* Acknowledge everything you've done to create a life you cherish.

More Chicken Soup?

Many of the stories and poems you have read in this book were submitted by readers like you who had read earlier *Chicken Soup for the Soul* books. We invite you to contribute a story to one of our future volumes.

Stories may be up to 1,200 words and must uplift or inspire. You may submit an original piece, something you have read or your favorite quotation on your refrigerator door.

To obtain a copy of our submission guidelines and a listing of upcoming *Chicken Soup* books, please write, fax or check our Web site.

Please send your submissions to:
Chicken Soup for the Soul
P.O. Box 30880
Santa Barbara, CA 93130, USA
fax: (001) 805-563-2945
Web site: *www.chickensoup.com*

Just send a copy of your stories and other pieces to the above address.

We will be sure that both you and the author are credited for your submission.

For information about speaking engagements, other books, audiotapes, workshops and training programs, please contact any of our authors directly.

Who Is Jack Canfield?

Jack Canfield is one of America's leading experts in the development of human potential and personal effectiveness. He is both a dynamic, entertaining speaker and a highly sought-after trainer. Jack has a wonderful ability to inform and inspire audiences toward increased levels of self-esteem and peak performance.

He is the author and narrator of several bestselling audio- and videocassette programs, including *Self-Esteem and Peak Performance, How to Build High Self-Esteem, Self-Esteem in the Classroom* and *Chicken Soup for the Soul—Live*. He is regularly seen on television shows such as *Good Morning America, 20/20* and *NBC Nightly News*. Jack has coauthored numerous books, including the *Chicken Soup for the Soul* series, *Dare to Win* and *The Aladdin Factor* (all with Mark Victor Hansen), *100 Ways to Build Self-Concept in the Classroom* (with Harold C. Wells), *Heart at Work* (with Jacqueline Miller) and *The Power of Focus* (with Les Hewitt and Mark Victor Hansen).

Jack is a regularly featured speaker for professional associations, school districts, government agencies, churches, hospitals, sales organizations and corporations. His clients have included the American Dental Association, the American Management Association, AT&T, Campbell's Soup, Clairol, Domino's Pizza, GE, ITT, Hartford Insurance, Johnson & Johnson, the Million Dollar Roundtable, NCR, New England Telephone, Re/Max, Scott Paper, TRW and Virgin Records. Jack has taught on the faculty of Income Builders International, a school for entrepreneurs.

Jack conducts an annual seven-day Training of Trainers program in the areas of self-esteem and peak performance. It attracts entrepreneurs, educators, counselors, parenting trainers, corporate trainers, professional speakers, ministers and others interested in developing their speaking and seminar-leading skills.

For further information about Jack's books, tapes and training programs, or to schedule him for a presentation, please contact:

Self-Esteem Seminars
P.O. Box 30880
Santa Barbara, CA 93130, USA
phone: (001) 805-563-2935 • fax: (001) 805-563-2945
Web site: *www.jackcanfield.com*

Who Is Mark Victor Hansen?

In the area of human potential, no one is better known and more respected than Mark Victor Hansen. For more than thirty years, Mark has focused solely on helping people from all walks of life reshape their personal vision of what's possible. His powerful messages of possibility, opportunity and action have helped create startling and powerful change in thousands of organizations and millions of individuals worldwide.

He is a sought-after keynote speaker, bestselling author and marketing maven. Mark's credentials include a lifetime of entrepreneurial success, in addition to an extensive academic background. He is a prolific writer with many bestselling books such as *The One Minute Millionaire, The Power of Focus, The Aladdin Factor* and *Dare to Win,* in addition to the *Chicken Soup for the Soul* series. Mark has also made a profound influence through his extensive library of audio programs, video programs and enriching articles in the areas of big thinking, sales achievement, wealth building, publishing success, and personal and professional development.

Mark is also the founder of MEGA Book Marketing University and Building Your MEGA Speaking Empire. Both are annual conferences where Mark coaches and teaches new and aspiring authors, speakers and experts on building lucrative publishing and speaking careers.

His energy and exuberance travel still further through mediums such as television *(Oprah, CNN* and *The Today Show),* print *(Time, U.S. News & World Report, USA Today, New York Times* and *Entrepreneur)* and countless radio and newspaper interviews as he assures our planet's people that *"you can easily create the life you deserve."*

As a passionate philanthropist and humanitarian, he's been the recipient of numerous awards that honor his entrepreneurial spirit, philanthropic heart and business acumen, including the prestigious Horatio Alger Award for his extraordinary life achievements, which stand as a powerful example that the free enterprise system still offers opportunity to all.

Mark Victor Hansen is an enthusiastic crusader of what's possible and is driven to make the world a better place.

Mark Victor Hansen & Associates, Inc.
P.O. Box 7665 • Newport Beach, CA 92658, USA
phone: (001) 949-764-2640 • fax: (001) 949-722-6912
FREE resources online at: *www.markvictorhansen.com*

Who Is Stephanie Marston?

Stephanie Marston is an internationally published author, acclaimed speaker and life-quality expert. She is the author of *If Not Now, When?*, *The Magic of Encouragement* and *The Divorced Parent*. Stephanie is also the creator of Chicken Soup's Life Coaching for Parents: Six Weeks to Sanity.

Stephanie is a licensed Marriage, Family Therapist with more than 25 years' experience in women's issues and parenting.

Ms. Marston has appeared on numerous radio and television programs such as *The Oprah Winfrey Show*, *The Early Show*, and *Women-to-Women*.

Stephanie is one of the most sought-after experts in the country offering her sage wisdom on a host of life-quality and family issues especially, how to balance life's competing priorities and create a high quality life. She has conducted seminars for more than 50,000 women, parents, and mental health professionals internationally.

Stephanie delivers keynote addresses, seminars and workshops to women's organizations, corporations, parent groups, professional conferences, association and the general public. Some of her clients have included Los Angeles Department of Water and Power, Chanel, The Young Presidents Organization, Union Bank, Northrop Corporation, ARCO Corporation, Paramount Studios, Cedar-Sinai Medical Center, Jackson Lewis Attorneys at Law, Parkville Hospital, WCI Communities and The Junior Leagues of America.

Whether you're a career woman struggling to balance the demands of work and family, a midlife woman trying to navigate this challenging transition, a frustrated parent who wants to create greater harmony in your home, or a woman who is simply tired of living an overloaded existence Stephanie Marston has the answers.

For further information about Stephanie's books, tapes and programs, or to schedule her for a presentation, please contact:

Life Quality Seminars
Box 31453
Santa Fe, New Mexico 87594-1453, USA
Phone: (001) 505-989-7596 • fax: (001) 505-989-4486
Web site: *www.stephaniemarston.com*

Contributors

Sherry Baker has written poetry and prose—and felt a deep connection to nature—all her life. She is still walking ecstatically through the splendor of West Coast Vancouver Island, and is working on her second book. Visit her Web site at *msn/groups/STARDREAMING* or e-mail her at *sherrym2@shaw.ca*.

Vickie Baker, a 1996 Amy Award recipient, suffered a near-fatal accident while flying, which left her a quadriplegic. She and her cat lived independently in Denver, Colorado. She worked as a freelance writer and cofacilitated a class on attendant care at Craig Hospital in Denver. She is the author of "On Wings of Joy" and "Surprised Hope." Vickie had a Bachelor of Science Degree in Business Administration and a Master of Social Work Degree. Vickie passed away on October 13, 2003.

Faith Andrews Bedford is the author of a number of art-history books and writes the "Kids in the Country" column for *Country Living*. She can be reach at *faithab@aol.com*.

Living in Mexico since the age of fifty, **Karen Blue** has written and published *Midlife Mavericks: Women Reinventing Their Lives in Mexico* and is co-publisher of a monthly Internet magazine, *Living at Lake Chapala* (*www.mexico-insights.com*). She also authors a monthly column, *Living in Mexico: From a Woman's Perspective* at *www.mexconnect.com*.

Isabel Bearman Bucher continues her love affair with life, her husband, children and friends. Her first book, *Nonro's Monkey: An Italian-American Memoir,* is still looking for a home. She and Robert enjoy exchanging homes throughout the world, marvel and praise their good health, and look with sympathetic understanding as their children and grandchildren find their way.

Maura J. Casey writes for *The Day,* a newspaper in New London, Connecticut. She has written for newspapers since 1983. Her columns have been published in more than fifty newspapers nationwide. She lives with her husband, Peter J. Panzarella, and two children, Anna and Tim, in rural Connecticut. She can be reached at *m.casey@theday.com.*

K. K. Choate was a housewife for twelve years before turning entrepreneur. "PTA Mom" is her first published work. A married mother of two, her stories are humorous, poignant and family-oriented. No matter your age or race, you'll find yourself and your family inside her essays. For more information, contact *KChoate874@aol.com.*

Mary Joe Clendenin earned her B.S. in education from Abilene Christian University; her M.S. in natural science from New Mexico Highlands University; her Education Specialist and Doctor of Education degrees from New Mexico State University. She writes a weekly column for the *Stephenville Empire Tribune* and has ten books in print. She can be reached at *www.our-town.com/clendenin* or *mjclen@our-town.com.*

Pamela Gilchrist Corson is a writer, inspirational speaker and president of PR~Link Public Relations. A communications pro with twenty years' experience, she coaches clients on messaging and marketing. She offers speaking and media-training seminars, is an award-winning magazine editor and teaches feature writing at Xavier University. Her speaking and writing help people build stronger relationships with Christ and each other. Pam lives in Cincinnati, Ohio, with her husband Glenn. She can be reached at (001) 513-233-9090 or *www.pamgilchrist.com.*

M. Regina Cram is a newspaper columnist and freelance writer. She writes an often humorous column about the challenges of weaving faith into everyday life, as well as a teen column for the Catholic news service. Regina lives with her husband and four teenagers, and can be reached at *r.cram@cox.net.*

After twenty-five years as an Air Force wife, **Twink DeWitt**—with her husband, Denny—served with Mercy Ships and Youth with a Mission. They founded Heritage Anchor to help others write the family stories that become legacies for future generations. Twink's passion is to see others improve their writing. She can be reached at *dewitt@tyler.net.*

Sue Diaz is an award-winning humor columnist, advertising copywriter, and author of *The Snake in the Spin Cycle: And Other Tales of Family Life*, a collection of essays. She also teaches an adult-education course called Write Your Life's Experiences. She can be reached at *www.suediaz.com.*

Karen C. Driscoll is mother to four young children. Her work has appeared in *Chicken Soup for the Mother & Daughter Soul, Chocolate for a Woman's Soul* series, *E-Pregnancy, Mothering Magazine, Brain-Child* and the anthology, *Toddler.* She can be reached at *KMHBRDRISCOLL@hotmail.com.*

Avis Drucker received her B.A in sociology, with high honors, and worked in corporate training. Retiring a "washashore" to Cape Cod, she's been published in *Primetime, The Aurorean, The Chronicle,* and received honorable mention for poetry in the *Writer's Digest* annual writing contest. She says, "Writing, traveling and family are the passions that fill my life."

Nancy B. Gibbs is a pastor's wife, a mother and grandmother. She is a weekly religion columnist and freelance writer. Nancy has been published in numerous *Chicken Soup for the Soul* books, along with hundreds of other publications. She is the author of four books. She can be reached at *Daiseydood@aol.com* or *www.nancybgibbs.com.*

Karen Fortner Granger is a freelance publicist, speaker and writer. She resides in South Florida with her husband, Eric. Information on speaking topics can be found at *www.karengranger.com.*

Stacey Granger has been writing essays about motherhood for ten years. Her other essays have appeared in previous *Chicken Soup for the Soul* books. Along with writing, Stacey is an award-winning photographer specializing in fine children's portraiture. She can be reached at *www.staceygranger.com.*

Louise Hamm, a retired administrator, started writing after retirement. She has had poems, business articles, and nonfiction stories published, including one in *Chicken Soup for the Kid's Soul* and another in *Chicken Soup for the Golden Soul.* She has three grown children and two grandsons.

Jennie Ivey is a former history teacher now working as a writer. She is a columnist for her local newspaper, writes magazine articles and stories, and is the author of *Tennessee Tales the Textbooks Don't Tell,* a collection of stories from Tennessee history. Jennie lives in Cookeville, Tennessee. She can be reached at *jivey@multipro.com.*

After raising her family, **June Cerza Kolf** spent twelve years doing hospice work and began her writing career. She has six published books relating to grief and terminal illness, and is a frequent contributor to inspirational magazines. Her most recent book, *Standing in the Shadow,* is for suicide survivors.

Patricia Lorenz, who enjoys all the nature she can cram into her busy writing/speaking life, is one of the top contributors to the *Chicken Soup for the Soul* books with stories in seventeen of them. She's the author of over 400 articles, a contributing writer for fifteen Daily Guideposts books, an award-winning columnist, and the author of four books. Her two latest, *Life's Too Short to Fold Your Underwear* and *Grab the Extinguisher, My Birthday Cake's on Fire* can be ordered through Guideposts Books at *www.dailyguideposts.com/store.* To contact Patricia for speaking opportunities: *patricialorenz@juno.com.*

Barbara McCloskey received her B.A. from the University of Wisconsin-Parkside, graduating magna cum laude in 1991. She lives happily with her husband, Ken, and cat, Vinnie, in her Wisconsin home. She has enjoyed writing since childhood, and will continue to explore this challenging and satisfying outlet for the rest of her life.

Kay Collier McLaughlin, Ph.D., holds a doctorate in counseling psychology from the Union Institute. Editor of the award-winning newspaper, *The Advocate,* she founded and heads Solo Flight, education and advocacy for single adults, and is a consultant, motivational speaker and leadership development trainer. She can be reached at *kcollierm@diolex.org.*

Karen McQuestion is a writer whose work has appeared in numerous publications, including *Newsweek,* the *Chicago Tribune* and the *Denver Post.* She resides in Hartland, Wisconsin, with her husband and three children.

Janet Lynn Mitchell is a wife, mother, author and inspirational speaker. She is the coauthor of *A Special Kind of Love, for Those Who Love Children with Special Needs,* published by Broadman and Holman, and Focus on the Family, 2004. Janet can be reached at *JanetLM@prodigy.net* or (fax) (001) 714-633-6309.

Carol McAdoo Rehme, one of *Chicken Soup*'s most prolific contributors, finds her niche—inspirational writing—is the perfect avenue for sharing life's lessons. As founding director of Vintage Voices, Inc., a nonprofit agency that provides engaging, interactive programs in eldercare facilities, she witnesses caregiving in its purest form: among the aged. She can be reached at *carol@rehme.com* or *www.rehme.com.*

A writer and educator, **Deborah M. Ritz** received her Bachelor of Arts from Dickinson College and Master of Teaching from University of Richmond. She facilitates creative writing workshops for children and teachers in Virginia, and has served as a writer-in-residence. Deborah is employed at the Virginia Museum of Fine Arts. She can be reached at *dr@moonlitwaters.com.*

Kris Hamm Ross is a teacher at Grace School in Houston, Texas. She is also a writer whose work has appeared in educational magazines, *The Houston Chronicle,* and other *Chicken Soup for the Soul* books. Her husband Matt, son Jay, and the fifth-graders she loves to teach, are frequent inspirations for the stories she writes. She can be reached at *klross@pdq.net.*

Myra Shostak is a writer and teacher with master's degres in child development and social work. She is the author of *Rainbow Candles: A Chanukah Counting Book.* Myra enjoys calligraphy, bookbinding, writing, quilting, working with children and learning new things. She can be reached at *MyraC345@msn.com.*

Deborah Shouse is a writer, editor and dreamer who believes in making the most of life's lessons. Her latest book is *Making Your Message Memorable: Communicating Through Stories.* Her work has appeared in *Spirituality & Health; Reader's Digest; Newsweek; Woman's Day; Family Circle* and *Ms.* Visit her Web site: *www.thecreativityconnection.com.*

Susan Siersma, mother of three, takes pleasure in reading, organic gardening and playing the violin. She also enjoys long walks with her husband, grandchildren and dog, Tipperary. The inspiration for Susan's writing comes from everyday life and the people around her. "Wisdom of the Birds" is dedicated to the memory of her father.

Sharla Taylor is a member of The National League of American Pen Women, Inc. She has contributed to *Chicken Soup for the Sister's Soul,* Expert Resumes for Health Care Careers and others. Read more of her writing online at: *www.sharlataylor.com < http://www.sharlataylor.com/>.* Her business Web site at *www.athomewithwords.com.* E-mail address: *athomewithwords@msn.com.*

Beverly Tribuiani-Montez, a freelance writer is currently living in Brentwood, California. She enjoys writing the 'truth,' in all its fragility. She believes everything is possible. Has a tattoo bearing her husband's name. Has a soft spot for teenagers. Admires those who are true to themselves and promotes education. She writes as a way of processing life and inspiring others. She can be reached at *bevie1967@aol.com*.

K. K. (Katherine Komninos) Wilder, a retired educator, makes her home in Burlington, Vermont, where she is a freelance writer and editor. Among other publications, her work appears in the *Don't Sweat Stories*. Her longtime column, "Disability Happens," earned her a Governor's Service Award in 2002.

Rita V. Williams is the executive director of a crisis pregnancy center in North Platte, Nebraska. Rita speaks regarding her class and the center services. North Platte is helping CardioJam get grants and exposure. She plans to help market the "I'm Watching It!" citywide health program. Cardiojam tapes sell for $10.00 each plus shipping. She can be reached at *riatwrc@kdsi.com*.

Susan Carver Williams is a freelance writer and editor, living in Durham, North Carolina. Her company, The Artful Word, specializes in content-development and layout and design of newsletters and collateral materials for small businesses and nonprofits. She is also the creator of Touchstones, one-of-a-kind personalized cookbooks, and other memory-maker gifts. She can be reached at *artfulword@nc.rr.com*.

Ferida Wolff is the author of *Listening Outside Listening Inside,* an inspirational book for adults, as well as sixteen books for children. She was both student and teacher of yoga for twenty-six years, and now facilitates meditation workshops. She can be reached at *www.feridawolff.com* or *fwolff@erols.com*.

Beadrin (Pixie) Youngdahl lives in Minnesota, where she works as a registered nurse, travels when the opportunity arises and reads almost any time she is not in motion (and sometimes when she is). She can be reached at *Beadrin@aol.com*.

Lynne Zielinski is a freelance writer in Huntsville, Florida. She believes that life is a gift from God and what we do with it is our gift *to* God. Lynne can be reached at *ARISWAY@aol.com*.

Permissions *(continued from page ii)*

Follow Your Heart. Reprinted by permission of Sherry Baker. ©2003 Sherry Baker.

View from an Empty Nest. Reprinted by permission of June Cerza Kolf. ©1992 June Cerza Kolf.

PTA Mom. Reprinted by permission of Kristy Choate. ©1997 Kristy Choate.

Taking the Leap. Reprinted by permission of Katherine Komninos Wilder. ©1988 Katherine Komninos Wilder.

Communing with Nature. Reprinted by permission of Nancy B. Gibbs. ©2003 Nancy B. Gibbs.

The Art of Saying "No." Reprinted by permission of Karen McQuestion. ©2001 Karen McQuestion.

Enjoying the Moment. Reprinted by permission of Stacey Granger. ©2000 Stacey Granger.

A Higher Education. Reprinted by permission of Barbara McCloskey. ©2003 Barbara McCloskey.

Parking in the Center of the Garage. Reprinted by permission of Louise R. Hamm. ©2001 Louise R. Hamm.

Feeling Free. Reprinted by permission of Ferida Wolff. ©1999 Ferida Wolff.

Life After Death. Reprinted by permission of Rita V. Williams. ©2001 Rita V. Williams.

If I Were Lucky. Reprinted by permission of Avis P. Drucker. ©2002 Avis P. Drucker.

Sticks and Stones. Reprinted by permission of Carol McAdoo Rehme. ©2002 Carol McAdoo Rehme.

The Dear Stand. Reprinted by permission of Jennie M. Ivey. ©2003 Jennie M. Ivey.

A Lasting Impression. Reprinted by permission of Sharla Taylor. ©2002 Sharla Taylor.

Granny's Ninth Birthday. Reprinted by permission of Lucie H. DeWitt. ©2002 Lucie H. DeWitt.

"Best" Truths and *The White Line.* Reprinted by permission of Isabel Bearman Bucher. ©2003 Isabel Bearman Bucher.

Knowing What Your Rope Is. Reprinted by permission of Myra C. Shostak. ©1988 Myra C. Shostak. Originally appeared in COPING - Winter 1988.